Springer Series on Medical Education

Steven Jonas, MD, Founding Editor
Carol J. Bland, PhD, Series Editor

2003   Medical Teaching in Ambulatory Care, 2nd ed, *Warren Rubenstein, MD, Yves Talbot, MD*

2002   Residents' Teaching Skills, *Janine C. Edwards, PhD, Joan A. Friedland, MD, MPH, and Robert Bing-You, MD, MEd, FACP, Editors*

2001   Fostering Reflection and Providing Feedback, Helping Others Learn from Experience,
Jane Westberg, PhD, with Hilliard Jason, MD, EdD

1996   Fostering Learning in Small Groups: A Practical Guide,
Jane Westberg, PhD, and Hilliard Jason, MD, EdD

1995   Innovators in Physician Education: The Process and Pattern of Reform at Ten North American Medical Schools,
Robert H. Ross, PhD, and Harvey V. Fineberg, MD, PhD

1994   Teaching Creatively with Video: Fostering Reflection, Communication and Other Clinical Skills,
Jane Westberg, PhD, and Hilliard Jason, MD, EdD

1993   Assessment Measures in Medical School, Residency, and Practice:
The Connections, *Joseph S. Gonnella, MD, Mohammadreza Hojat, PhD, James B. Erdmann, PhD, and J. Jon Veloski, MS*

1992   Collaborative Clinical Education: The Foundation of Effective Health Care,
Jane Westberg, PhD, and Hilliard Jason, MD, EdD

1992   Medical Teaching in Ambulatory Care: A Practical Guide,
Warren Rubenstein, MD, and Yves Talbot, MD

1989   Successful Faculty in Academic Medicine: Essential Skills and
How to Acquire Them, *Carole J. Bland, PhD, Constance C. Schmitz, MA, Frank T. Stritter, PhD, Rebecca C. Henry, PhD, and John J. Aluise, PhD*

1988   A Practical Guide to Clinical Teaching in Medicine,
Kaaren C. Douglas, MD, MSPH, Michael C. Hosokawa, EdD, and Frank H. Lawler, MD, MSPH

1987   Clinical Teaching for Medical Residents: Roles, Techniques, and Programs,
Janine C. Edwards, PhD, and Robert L. Marier, MD, FACP, Editors

1985   Implementing Problem-Based Curriculum for the Preclinical Years,
Howard S. Barrows, MD, FRCP (C)

1985   How to Design a Problem-Based Curriculum for the Preclinical Years,
Howard S. Barrows, MD,

1982   The Art of Teaching Primary Care, *Archie S. Golden, MD, MPH, Dennis G. Carlson, MD, MPH, MA, and Jan L. Hagen, MSW, Editors*

1980   Problem-Based Learning: An Approach to Medical Education,
Howard S. Barrows, MD, and Robyn M. Tamblyn, BScN

Warren Rubenstein, MD, is a family physician trained in medical education at the Family Medicine Programme, Royal College of General Practitioners of Australia. He is assistant professor in the Department of Family and Community Medicine at the University of Toronto. Since 1978, he has taught medical students and residents in his office at Mount Sinai Hospital in Toronto, where he recently completed his tenure as family physician-in-chief.

Yves Talbot, MD, is a family physician whose primary work in medical education is with faculty development. He is professor in the Departments of Family and Community Medicine and Health Administration at the University of Toronto and teaches at Mount Sinai Hospital, Toronto. Formerly the director of research, he is currently the director of international programs. He has been working in South America since 1995, conducting training programs to develop primary care. He has a particular interest in the role of primary care and health equity.

Medical Teaching in Ambulatory Care

Second Edition

Warren Rubenstein, MD
Yves Talbot, MD

 Springer Publishing Company

Springer Publishing Company, Inc.
536 Broadway
New York, NY 10012-3955

Acquisitions Editor: Sheri W. Sussman
Production Editor: Janice G. Stangel
Cover design by Joanne Honigman

03 04 05 06 07 / 5 4 3 2 1

Library of Congress Cataloging-in-Publication Data

Rubenstein, Warren.
  Medical teaching in ambulatory care / Warren Rubenstein, Yves Talbot. — 2nd ed.
      p. ; cm. — (Springer series on medical education)
  Includes bibliographical references and index.
  ISBN 0-8261-7691-7
    1. Ambulatory medical care—Study and teaching.   I. Talbot, Yves.   II. Title.   III. Springer series on medical education (Unnumbered)
  [DNLM: 1. Ambulatory Care.   2. Education, Medical, Graduate—methods.   3. Teaching—methods.   WX 18 R896m 2003]
  R834.R83 2003
  610'.71'55—dc21   2003041616

Printed in the United States of America by Sheridan Books.

To Susan and Jonathan—carpe diem.
WR

To my father, Roland, my wife, Lois and my sons,
Adam and Martin—who are my teachers
YT

Contents

Acknowledgments

The authors would like to thank the following who so graciously aided in the evolution of this book: Dr. David Tannenbaum, for the groundwork in Chapter 3; Dr. Larry Librach, for the framework of Chapter 6; Dr. Brian Goldman, for the first edit of the original manuscript; Dr. Allan Rosenbluth, for the psychiatric profiles in Chapter 5; Dr. Richard Tiberius, whose workshops with Dr. Rubenstein provided the basis for Chapter 2; Dr. Helen Batty, for advice on educational theory; Joanne Permaul and Rita Shaughnessy, for library research; staff members of the Image Center, Mount Sinai Hospital, for graphics; Susan Devins, for getting difficult concepts into plain English; Drs. Anne Biringer, June Carroll, and David Tannenbaum, our colleagues at Mount Sinai Hospital, with whom we have discussed and developed many of these ideas; Drs. Wes Fabb, Peter Fleming, and Michael Heffernan, for their guiding light; and the Dr. Barnet and Beverley Giblon Professorship in Family and Community Medicine at the University of Toronto for academic support.

Introduction

FOR WHOM THE AUTHORS TOILED— A SECOND TIME

The first edition of this book has been widely used by physicians who teach medical students or residents in ambulatory care. Both primary care physicians and specialists have been the audience. Historically, physicians in ambulatory hospital-based teaching units and associated outpatient clinics were the locus for trainee assignment. Many residency programs own and/or manage an ambulatory clinic for their trainees, within a hospital or in its vicinity. More recently, community-based locations have been widely used. This refers to the practice office, solo or group, where the practitioner is the physician of record for, and provides continuity of care to, the patients (Deutsch, 1997). In addition to these community practitioners' offices, staff-model health maintenance organizations and community health centers also serve as teaching centers. Trainees are also now found in ambulatory surgery centers, family planning clinics, urgent care centers, public health offices, and student health services.

This book outlines the knowledge and skills of teaching that will assist you in working with residents and medical students. It does not tell you the content of ambulatory care, that is, not what to teach, but suggests approaches to teaching that can be applied in the context of various specialties for the needs of a particular learner. The goals and content of ambulatory teaching experiences may be different across specialties, but the teaching skills are mostly generic (Biddle, Siska, & Erney, 1994). As you change from bedside teaching to deskside teaching, it will give you the tools to make you and your ambulatory setting an effective educational milieu.

WHY AMBULATORY CARE TEACHING?

Since this book's first edition, there has been a consolidation of the paradigm shift (Kuhn, 1970) from hospital-based patient care to ambulatory care (Stearns & Glasser, 1993). As a result of economic forces and advances in health care delivery, many acute illnesses and exacerbations of chronic diseases are managed effectively without hospitalization (Green, Fryer, Yawn, Lanier, & Dovey, 2001). Many medical and surgical subspecialties can now be practiced almost exclusively in the outpatient setting. The case mix on many inpatient services has shifted dramatically. Beds are filled with critically ill patients requiring specialized care, with patients hospitalized transiently, or with those who have had an extensive preadmission workup. These patients are rarely suitable for teaching medical students or residents (Deutsch, 1997; Kassirer, 1996; Prideaux & Alexander, 2000).

Three decades ago, training programs in family practice recognized that most of the work of family physicians was in office-based settings, and only a fraction of their time was spent in hospitals. This led to the development of model training practices in hospitals and the use of private offices in surrounding communities (Link & Buchsbaum, 1986). Soon after, general internal medicine (Wones, Rouan, Brody, Bode, & Radack, 1986) and general pediatrics followed suit. Then there arose limited training in other specialties (Levy, 1988) and a call for ambulatory training in the general undergraduate curriculum (Panel on the GPEP, 1984; Shine, 1986). Per-koff's seminal article in 1986 alerted the world of medical education that it was time to move trainees to the settings where the patients could be found with the common problems about which they should be learning (Perkoff, 1986).

Over the past 10 years, there has been an explosion of ambulatory care teaching programs. Almost every medical discipline has at least part of its residency training in ambulatory sites. Many clinical clerkships, both primary care and specialty, include a significant component of ambulatory experience (Lynch, Whitley, Basnight, & Patselas, 1999). Even introductory clinical courses taught in the preclinical years have made use of ambulatory settings (Steward, 1993). There has been an endless stream of journal papers, both descriptive and research, about these programs (Bowen & Irby, 2002; Irby, 1995; Kilminster & Jolly, 2000; Heidenreich, Lye, Simpson, & Lourich, 2000). There are several textbooks (Deutch, 1997; Whitehouse, Roland, & Campion, 1997) providing more in-depth program descriptions. This book is one of the few "how to" guides to help you with your teaching skills.

FROM HOSPITAL TO AMBULATORY CARE TEACHING

Inpatient teaching is quite familiar to all of us. A medical student or resident admits patients, either electively or as an emergency. They perform a detailed history and physical, and they formulate a differential diagnosis and a treatment plan. The latter are shaped by initial discussion with a more senior trainee and then a more detailed round with an attending physician at a designated time. Formal housestaff teaching—aside from the teaching required to help the trainee deal with the patient's problems requiring immediate treatment—is left for later. In the early years of the undergraduate curriculum, students spend an hour or more at the bedside of a hospitalized patient doing a history and physical. There follows a lengthy review with teacher and fellow group members beside the captive patient.

In ambulatory settings, one-to-one teaching occurs most often directly after the patient is seen, simultaneously with patient care. Sometimes, immediate problems are dealt with exclusively. Or, the patient may be presenting for ongoing care of a long-term illness. Ambulatory patients are there for a short period and, because they are not acutely ill, exercise more control as to what happens to them (Schwenk & Whitman, 1987). There are significant time pressures on teachers and their medical students or residents. The need to see patients in a cost-efficient manner increases the burden on teachers to review cases rapidly (Skeff, 1988). This book focuses on teaching in this context.

GUIDEBOOK TO AMBULATORY CARE TEACHING

The authors have worked for 25 years in ambulatory care teaching and base this book on that experience. We have reflected on what works and what does not, which theories are practical and which are not.

This book follows the personal development of "Dr. Z. Z. Smith" as a teacher and the transformation of his multispecialty clinic to a teaching center. Shortly after establishing his practice, Dr. Smith, a representative of all specialties, finds that students and residents from the local hospital in which he does rounds are asking to come to his office. Without any previous teacher training, he naturally has difficulty with the daily challenges of these learners. He sets out to see if he can learn more about being a teacher.

In chapter 1, we will, with Dr. Smith, explore basic educational theory. He finds theories that provide him with a more formal framework for his teaching rather than his old style of improvising. Among the theories he discovers are reception and discovery learning (contrasting approaches to presenting information), adult learning (a set of guidelines to treat trainees as mature learners), and contract learning (a method of helping students to define what and how they will learn).

In chapter 2, we will follow Dr. Smith as he looks into specific teaching skills. He finds out that teachers go through a two-step process at each encounter before reaching the teaching point. They choose a learner premise (based on their observations of the trainee) or a teacher premise (based on their previous experience with trainees in general) and then use a specific teaching skill in that circumstance. Dr. Smith discovers a variety of teaching skills within three umbrella categories—telling, asking, and showing—and becomes familiar with the situations in which each would be most useful.

In chapter 3, Dr. Smith enlists his colleagues to use the entire clinic as a teaching center. This process requires preparation of the office itself, the patients, and the medical office staff for teaching in the clinic. The examining rooms must be made ready for teaching. Brochures and posters are needed to inform the patients about the clinic's new teaching role. The office staff are involved in planning for the students' arrival and determine that they can play a role in the students' learning. Finally, the medical staff set up their own meeting to learn about their teaching role. The steady inflow of trainees to the clinic pressures the medical staff to develop some teaching strategies to use during the workday. In chapter 4, the staff learn about case discussion using the patients' presenting problems for immediate discussion with the students, and case review, a strategy for teaching with these cases later in the day. They consider the advantages and disadvantages of using the patients' charts for teaching. They also analyze such techniques as role play and didactic presentations.

One year later, Dr. Smith and his colleagues find that they have some difficult trainees in their clinic who tax their teaching abilities. In chapter 5, the staff see how to gather the group together to develop strategies for helping students with problems in clinical learning such as poor knowledge base or difficulty in making clinical judgments. They seek mechanisms to assist learners who are prejudiced or who avoid the difficult patient. They devise a system to help other students who are argumentative or defensive. In addition, they tackle the troublesome matter of learners' personal problems, such as overconfidence, lying, and drug abuse.

The core of chapter 6 is evaluation, a three-pronged approach that shows how Dr. Smith evaluates his trainees, his teachers, and the clinic's teaching program. An overview of evaluation theory leads to a sample of rating forms in which students evaluate the teachers, students evaluate the office as a teaching center, and the teachers in turn evaluate the students.

This is a guide to using your office as an important locus of medical education. It will assist those teaching graduate trainees, clinical clerks, and medical students on electives as well as those teaching undergraduate students in core topics.

The future of medical education is in ambulatory care teaching.

REFERENCES

Biddle, B., Siska, K., & Erney, S. (1994). A description of ambulatory teaching in a longitudinal primary care program. *Teaching and Learning in Medicine, 6,* 185–190.

Bowen, J., & Irby, D. (2002). Assessing quality and costs of education in ambulatory settings: A review of the literature. *Academic Medicine, 77,* 621–680.

Deutsch, S. (1997). *Community-based teaching.* Philadelphia: American College of Physicians.

Green, L., Fryer, G., Yawn, B., Lanier, D., & Dovey, S. (2001). The ecology of medical care revisited. *New England Journal of Medicine, 344,* 2021–2025.

Heidenreich, C., Lye, P., Simpson, D., & Lourich, M. (2000). The search for effective and efficient ambulatory teaching methods through the literature. *Pediatrics, 105,* 231–237.

Irby, D. (1995). Teaching and learning in ambulatory settings: A thematic review of the literature. *Academic Medicine, 70,* 898–930.

Kassirer, J. (1996). Redesigning graduate medical education—location and content. *New England Journal of Medicine, 335,* 507–509.

Kilminster, S., & Jolly, B. (2000). Effective clinical supervision in clinical practice settings: A literature review. *Medical Education, 34,* 827–840.

Kuhn, T. S. (1970). *The structure of scientific revolutions.* Chicago: The University of Chicago Press.

Levy, M. (1988). An ambulatory program for surgical residents and medical students. *Journal of Medical Education, 63,* 386–391.

Link, K., & Buchsbaum, D. (1986). An agenda for residency training in ambulatory care. *Journal of Medical Education, 59,* 494–500.

Lynch, D., Whitley, T., Basnight, L., & Patselas, T. (1999). Comparison of ambulatory and inpatient experiences in five specialties. *Medical Teacher, 6,* 594–596.

Panel on the General Professional Education of the Physician. (1984). Physicians for the twenty-first century: The GPEP report. *Journal of Medical Education, 59,* 1–208.

Perkoff, G. (1986). Teaching clinical medicine in the ambulatory setting: An idea whose time may have finally come. *New England Journal of Medicine, 314,* 27–31.

Prideaux, D., & Alexander, H. (2000). Clinical teaching: Maintaining an educational role for doctors in the new health care environment. *Medical Education, 34,* 820–826.

Schwenk, T. L., & Whitman, N. (1987). *The physician as teacher.* Baltimore: Williams & Wilkin.

Shine, K. (1986). Innovations in ambulatory care education. *New England Journal of Medicine, 314,* 52–53.

Skeff, K. (1988). Enhancing teaching effectiveness and vitality in the ambulatory setting. *Journal of General Internal Medicine, 3,* S26–S33.

Stearns, J., & Glasser, M. (1993). How ambulatory care is different: A paradigm for teaching and practice. *Medical Education, 27,* 35–40.

Steward, D. (1993). Moving medical education out of the hospital. *Teaching and Learning in Medicine, 5,* 214–216.

Whitehouse, C., Roland, M., & Campion, P. (1997). *Teaching medicine in the community.* Oxford: Oxford University Press.

Wones, R., Rouan, G., Brody, T., Bode, R., & Radack, K. (1986). An ambulatory medical education program for internal medicine residents. *Journal of Medical Education, 314,* 27–31.

—1—

Learning and Teaching in Ambulatory Care

Dr. Z. Z. Smith completed his residency 5 years ago and began working with a large multispecialty clinic. Like many of his colleagues, he admitted patients to the local teaching hospital and taught the medical students and housestaff on a daily basis. Soon, because of his enthusiasm, trainees asked him if they could see patients with him in his office.

Dr. Smith enjoyed teaching and was pleased that students were interested in coming to his office. Like some doctors, however, he had no training in teaching and felt that his teaching skills were inadequate. He wondered why some teaching sessions were successful and others were not. In addition, when problems arose, he had no concept of how to handle them. He decided to read some education textbooks to find learning theory that could be useful to his teaching with trainees in his office. A set of principles would help him improve his trainees' learning and assist him in dealing with the frustrations that he encountered as a teacher.

Seven subjects attracted his interest:

1. Learning
2. Teaching
3. Adult learning
4. Content and process learning
5. Reflection
6. Domains of learning
7. Contract learning

The following sections discuss what he learned about these terms.

1

LEARNING

There are two ways that the teacher can present information to the learner (Ausubel, 1968).

   1.   *Reception learning:* The entire content of what is to be learned is presented in its final form. (Example: A complete set of notes about family planning is handed out to medical students at the start of their ambulatory gynecology rotation.)
   2.   *Discovery learning:* The content of what is to be learned is based on exploration and questioning by the student using her existing knowledge. (Example: Instead of having a complete set of notes handed out, a seminar is held at the start of the gynecology rotation in which the students discuss the areas of family planning about which they need to know more and then plan how they will find out that information for themselves.)

A widely used example of discovery learning is problem-based learning, now extensively used in undergraduate medical curricula (Schatz, 1993). Students are given a written patient, health-delivery, or research problem as a stimulus for learning. Students tackle problems in small groups under the supervision of a tutor (Barrows & Tamblyn, 1980; Boud & Feletti, 1999). In chapter 4, find out how you can use problem-based learning in your office.

Reception learning saves time for the teacher. It is an efficient method for presenting large amounts of material to be learned (Ausubel, 1968). The information is well-organized for the learner, who then usually memorizes the facts and stores the details in long-term memory.

Discovery learning takes more time for both student and teacher, but makes the learning more interesting and challenging. Knowledge acquired by discovery is more likely to be remembered, more available for recall, and more likely to be applied in novel situations (Bruner, 1968). But, the information tends to be initially gathered in a disorganized series of facts. The teacher needs to help the learner to organize their memory by drawing links to specific cases, or using mnemomic organizers, e.g., the ABC's of resuscitation (Bordage, 1994). Discovery learning also encourages independent study and thus the acquisition of learning skills that will be useful for continuing education when one is practice, especially Internet-based knowledge management (Evans, 2001).

TEACHING

Of the differing definitions of teaching (Joyce & Weil, 1992), we find that the most useful one is: Teaching is the facilitation of learning. The teacher acts as a guide or helper, not as the giver of knowledge or spoon-feeder (Tough, 1971).

Learning is a shared process between teacher and learner, and not just the responsibility of the teacher. The teacher's role is to challenge the trainee by alerting him to the problem at hand. This is also known as "creating the need to know." Students who recognize the need to know expend more learning effort, are superior at reformulating new information and applying it to their own setting, are able to combine better new material with existing knowledge to ensure long-term learning, and devote more time to practice and review (Ausubel, 1968).

The trainee may not always be aware of the issues to be learned, and the teacher should try to highlight these for them. For example, the topic of practice management may be one of the objectives of the ambulatory block. A resident may not realize the importance of this topic or even fathom what she needs to learn in this subject. One might "create the need to know" by asking the resident to spend an hour or two at the reception desk talking to patients, answering the telephone, and making appointments. From this experience, the resident learns the complexities of an office and realizes that she has much to learn about practice management. The resident can then be motivated to indicate what she or he specifically wants to learn. The result is a captivated learner.

It is also part of the teacher's job to recognize and use teachable moments. The time immediately following an interaction between trainee and patient is a valuable one for learning (Whitman & Magill, 2000). The impact of a teaching point related to that clinical encounter, while it is fresh in the trainee's mind, can make a lasting impression. There are particularly special moments, such as following an emotionally charged visit or a challenging diagnostic problem, when long-term learning could be further enhanced.

For example, a resident reports that he is seeing Mrs. Jones, who arrived at the office without an appointment and wanted to be seen because of chest pain. The resident notes from the chart that the patient has been seen several times for chest pain and that each time it was diagnosed as chest wall pain. After a brief history, he concludes that the pain is not serious and wants to tell the patient to return if it recurs. When you see the patient, however, you discover that the patient has been awakened at night by this pain, almost daily this past week. You do an electrocardiogram and see S-T segment elevations in the lateral leads. The patient is sent to the emergency department at your local hospital. Afterward, you use the moment to discuss with the resident the importance of a thorough history when seeing patients with chest pain.

PRINCIPLES OF ADULT LEARNING

In grade school, students learn according to the principles of pedagogy. Pedagogy assumes that the learner is dependent, teacher centered, with little previous knowledge, and ready to learn what he is told. Students continue to learn in this manner throughout most of their schooling experience, including the first years of medical school. The physician, like all adults, learns differently, however (MacKeracher, 1996; Brookfield, 1990).

For example, think of a colleague who wants to learn furniture refinishing. He buys a dining room table in poor condition. Instead of having it refinished by a contractor, he decides to save some money by doing it himself. He reads some books and magazines and consults with experts. He works at it in his spare time on weekends. He completes the job himself by trial and error as well as by learning from comments from his spouse. The table now sits in the dining room.

Let us try to learn some principles from your colleague's experience.

1. He was ready to learn when a perceived need was there (the table was bought, it was in bad shape, and it was too expensive to send out).
2. He selected his own learning experiences (books and advice rather than a course at the local school).
3. It was a problem-oriented task (table in terrible shape).
4. He applied his new skills and knowledge immediately (he went from book to working on the table).
5. He obtained evaluation as to his progress (trial and error, from his spouse's comments, and how it looked to him, i.e., self-evaluation).

There are two additional principles of adult learning.

1. The learner thrives in a nonthreatening learning environment.
2. The learner strives to contribute from his own reservoir of knowledge and skills to help others.

The principles of adult learning are known as andragogy (Barer-Stein & Kompf, 2001). Medical students and residents primarily learn by using pedagogic skills from their previous 15 years of schooling. Having grown into adulthood, however, they now have andragogic expectations. We call this a pedandragogic learner: a child in an adult shell. The learner has the expectations of an adult but possesses only the learning skills of a child.

Essential to adult learning is trainees defining their own learning objectives. A learning objective is a statement of what the trainee should be able to do at the end of his course (Fabb, Heffernan, Phillips, & Stone, 1976). Well-defined objectives are helpful to both teacher and trainee, so that both are clear on what is being attempted in the learning situation.

Learning objectives should be very specific, defined in terms of the behavior of the learner not the teacher, based on the needs of the learner, and achievable in the time allotted (Miller, 1962). Here is an example of some objectives for a third-year student coming to an ophthalmology office for a one-week rotation.

At the end of this elective, the student will be able to do the following:

- List the differential diagnosis of the red eye
- Use the ophthalmoscope to identify a cataract
- Know the drugs used to dilate the pupil

Formulating learning objectives is a joint activity for teacher and learner. The ultimate list will be based on a combination of the objectives of the course, your previous experience with learners at a similar level of training, and the learner's own identified needs (Mager, 1962).

Medical trainees find it difficult to define their own learning objectives because teachers have always told them what is to be learned. They also have difficulty defining learning strategies for themselves because the strategies have always been set out in advance. The trainees assume they have little knowledge of their own because they have always been treated that way. When expected to contribute and base learning on knowledge they probably have, they find it distressing. They fear receiving progress reports because, up until now, evaluation has always been a negative, authoritarian experience rather than a step in assisting learning. Finally, they cannot accept teachers as colleagues because they have always seen teachers as authoritarian (Rogers, 1983).

Keep this conflict in mind when planning your teaching, for when you try to apply the principles of adult learning to your trainees, at first they may not be able to operate under these principles because they have never learned how to act as adult learners. You may need to take the time to explain how to be an adult learner while they unlearn the learning habits of their previous schooling (Knowles, 1975). It will be time well spent, for the skills they learn will be the ones they need to use as graduate doctors after training. Then they are on their own to define gaps in knowledge, to keep up on new knowledge, and to determine for themselves how they will learn this material.

Here is an example of how to apply the principles of adult learning to teaching in your ambulatory setting. When trainees first arrive in your office, discuss the areas in which they feel the need for more experience. Help them to identify these areas by reviewing their training to date. Explore topics that have kindled some special interest. Inquire about knowledge gaps they may have recognized. Prompt them by presenting a list of common conditions seen in your office, so that they can then select cases for which they need more experience. (Learn when a perceived need exists.) Together you can plan their work schedule, decide which patients they should see, identify whom else they might consult to learn certain topics, and determine suggested readings (they prefer to select their learning strategies). They can begin seeing patients that day to highlight some of those issues (they problem solving, immediate application). Then make an agreement to review their performance after a specific period (they want to know their progress).

CONTENT AND PROCESS LEARNING

The following two theories provide complementary approaches to learning, choosing the most effective and efficient strategy for the circumstance:

1. *Content learning:* The learner is presented with established facts and knowledge in a prescribed format with predetermined objectives. Elementary schools use this method frequently. Students are presented with books and classroom instruction and with tests based on the predetermined material. It is the least expensive method of instruction for large groups, when resources or time is limited, or when a large body of material needs to be covered. It is appropriate for learning factual information such as details of symptoms and signs of illness, investigations and treatments, laboratory interpretation, and therapeutics (Biggs, 1973).

2. *Process learning:* According to this theory of learning, we learn from what we do (Dewey, 1938). The knowledge and information for learning comes from what is happening in the environment in which the trainee is working (McLuhan, 1964, 1967). The work setting and

what teachers and trainees do there can make a lasting impression on the learner (Postman & Weingartner, 1969). The environment in which the trainee is working can provide the learning material (Bruner, 1960) as a contrast to a list of facts that is presented for learning.

As an example, you may never have a seminar on charting for the residents rotating through your pediatric office. Each of your charts, however, has an opening sheet that summarizes all the patient's medical problems, immunizations, developmental milestones, and medications. At each patient review, the resident updates the front sheet. For each new patient, the resident completes the front sheet. In addition, the resident sees that your coworkers also complete the summary sheet at each visit and constantly refer to it when first seeing a patient or when seeing a patient for a colleague on holiday. This resident learns very well the use and value of chart summary sheets and, from our experience, better than could ever be explained in a seminar.

Thus process learning is an appropriate method for learning attitudes and skills that cannot be easily transmitted as factual information. The skilled teacher will be knowledgeable about both content and process learning and choose one depending on topic, resources, and student.

REFLECTION

The concept of reflection is a helpful theme for teachers of medical trainees. When learners rush from one activity to another, they are at risk of mindlessly repeating bad habits and failing to learn from their experiences (Westberg & Jason, 1994). Reflection is an ongoing process of evaluating, interpreting, and deliberating (Smith & Irby, 1997; Schwartz & Bone, 1995). Reflective observation involves viewing a new experience through the interpretive lens of prior experience, current readings, and the teacher's assistance.

Seminal thinking about reflection in professionals' education came from Schon (Schon, 1987). In those professions that combine academic learning with practical work, certain individuals are identifiably more excellent than the majority. Through a series of empirical studies, Schon found that these outstanding practitioners consistently reflected on their work in such a way as they continually learned from it. This model of reflection represents an ideal for doctors and thus is appropriate in medical education.

Schon describes the practitioner as working with knowledge-in-action. This is the bank of information and skills learned over the years from school, books, journals, and experience. This knowledge is deeply embedded and often used automatically, without thinking about it. A simple example is riding a bike. In medicine, skilled physicians often recognize a particular disease the moment the affected individual walks in the door or relates the first few symptoms. Usually this knowledge-in-action gets the doctor through the day. But sometimes a familiar routine produces an unexpected result, or an error resists correction. As Schon states, this "surprise" happens when something fails to meet expectations. In an attempt to preserve constancy of the usual patterns of knowledge, the doctor may respond to surprise by brushing it aside, selectively not attending to the signals that produce it.

Better yet, the doctor will stop and think (reflection-in-action), which gives rise to an on-the-spot experiment. She will think up and try out new actions, questions, or diagnoses and observe the result. The experiment, if successful on a few occasions (reflection-on-action), will then become part of the new knowledge base.

Schon encourages the teacher to coach the student at each step of the reflection process (see Fig. 1.1).

Knowledge-in-Action: This is the trainee's knowledge base, which you will assess on an ongoing basis as you interact around cases. Where deficiencies are recognized, encourage self-directed reading; offer articles, books,

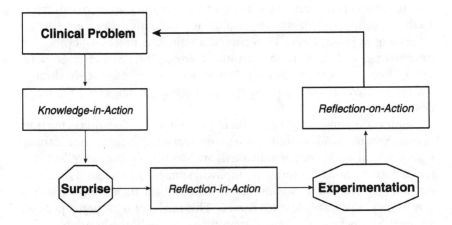

FIGURE 1.1 The reflection process.

or websites available in your office; or assign a learning project. (There are more specific ideas in chapters 2 and 4.)

Surprise: Support recognition of moments in clinical practice when the trainee notes variation from the usual. Engage in a dialogue about these clinical problems and about how they differ from the norm. Within your specialty, help trainees respect the concept of prevalence. Some diagnoses will be most common, but awareness of a larger breadth of diagnostic possibilities will prevent premature closure—the tendency to stop asking questions or asking questions to make a diagnosis fit. You can create "surprise" in your teaching by asking "what if . . . "—what if this 32-year-old female with shortness of breath was on oral contraceptives?

Reflection-in-Action/Experimentation: Upon recognizing a "surprise," encourage the trainee to rethink her knowledge base in ways that go beyond the usual rules, facts, and theories. Make the learning environment in your office one that encourages risk taking, thinking aloud, and discussing alternative perspectives. Remind the learner of her previous experimentation in similar circumstances. Send the trainee back in with the patient to test a new strategy. Invite students to keep journals of insights gained or questions raised and discuss these at a later time. Also, model the reflective process by relating examples from your own patients that day.

> "I saw a young female athlete today with a painful ankle sprain. She was so distraught. I assumed she was in so much pain, that I offered additional analgesia. She declined and just cried. I realized that I had missed the point here and then asked her what was upsetting her so much. She then related how this injury would cause her to miss the championship tournament, a goal for which she had been working for so long."

DOMAINS OF LEARNING

A domain of learning is a grouping of educational objectives into a distinctly limited area of knowledge. When learning objectives are grouped, they can be referred to with greater precision. They may help teachers and learners avoid confusion about what each has in mind for learning. Through reference to domains of learning, teachers and trainees should be better able to define nebulous objectives and discover a wider range of topics for a trainee's ambulatory experience. For example, in listing the objectives for an elective, teacher and trainee may find that all the objectives fall into a certain domain. By thinking about other domains, they could include a broader range of objectives (Mackway-Jones & Walker, 1999).

Topics covered in an ambulatory setting fit into one of three domains of learning.

1. *Cognitive domain:* Those objectives that deal with the recall or recognition of factual knowledge (Bloom, Englehart, Furst, Hill, & Krathwohl, 1956), such as:

    • Differential diagnosis of jaundice
    • Medical treatment of endometriosis
    • Pathology of tumors of the kidney

2. *Affective domain:* Those objectives that describe verbal skills, language, attitudes, and values (Krathwohl, Bloom, & Masia, 1964), such as:

    • Interviewing skills
    • Interaction with dying patients
    • Physician's stress management

3. *Psychomotor domain:* Those objectives listing technical and procedural skills, such as:

    • Ophthalmoscopy
    • Skin closure
    • Nasal packing

When teaching a particular topic, it is helpful to know in which domain that topic fits. A certain teaching skill may be more suited for one domain of learning than another (see Chapter 4).

LEARNING CONTRACTS

The use of learning contracts, which can be applied to teaching in the ambulatory setting, is based on adult learning theory. Contract learning is a process whereby trainees develop some of their own learning objectives, learning strategies, and evaluation methods that will be particular to their own needs and previous experience (Boak, 1998).

Contract learning has several advantages. Sharing responsibility for learning with the trainee may help make teaching less frustrating. It assists you in dealing with the widely varying backgrounds and previous experience, interests, learning styles, and learning speeds that students bring to your practice. Teachers usually cope with the variety by "aiming at the middle," hoping that those not quite ready for the teaching point will catch up later and those ahead of it will not get too bored. In addition, different learners interpret generic course objectives differently and may have little sense of ownership of the objectives.

In contract learning, given the trainee's needs and abilities and the time available, you and the trainee define learning objectives. By establishing his or her own objectives, the learner is more likely to understand them and to have more of a sense of personal commitment to them. Finally, in this process, you are not responsible solely for identifying how the learner will be able to accomplish all the objectives defined. When asked, the learner often discovers a richer variety of resources that are particularly related to his or her learning style.

There is a more long-term goal for the use of contract learning. For trainees, there is never enough time to learn everything in your specialty. It is always more than could ever be learned in the time allotted. When trainees leave the supervised medical learning environment, they are on their own to learn the rest and keep up on changes. By going through the process of contract learning, you will give the trainee some practice at the skills of lifelong learning—identifying weaknesses, setting learning objectives, and designing appropriate learning strategies.

You can use learning contracts in two ways. If you have the time and resources, you can use the formal method described here. In some cases, however, a more abbreviated version of the same concept is still valuable.

1. *Formal contract learning:* In this process, you formulate with the learner a written plan according to the structured sheet shown in Table 1.1. With your help, learners define their objectives and select various learning resources (in addition to the patients in your office)—books, articles, videos, seminars, and so forth. You set a completion date and agree on an evaluation method.

2. *Learning list:* Here you apply the principles of contract learning in a modified version. As in the formal method, you agree on learning objectives and write them down in a list. Thus you and the trainee have a list of key items that learners would like to accomplish during their stay. Review the list so that the objectives are drawn from a combination of cognitive, affective, and psychomotor domains. Both you and the trainee should keep a copy of the list. Refer to the list during and at

TABLE 1.1   Learning Contract

| Learner: Z. Z. Smith | | Rotation: General Surgery |
| Supervisor: Z. Z. Smith | | Date: January 1, 20XX |

Objectives	Resources	Evaluation
Learn removal of cysts	Clinic MDs Course at hospital (January 10)	Perform excision under supervision (January 31)
Treatment of burns	Clinic MDs Clinic nurses Library reading	Present burn management at clinic meeting (January 22)
Wound care after leaving hospital	Patients Clinic MDs Clinic nurses Home care nurses (make some visits)	Short oral quiz by supervisor (January 25)

the conclusion of the rotation to see whether you are meeting the objectives. Sometimes, the objectives need to be changed. Periodic meetings help the trainee and teacher keep the objectives in mind.

REFERENCES

Ausubel, D. (1968). *Educational psychology—A cognitive view.* New York: Holt, Rinehart.
Barer-Stein, T., & Kompf, M. (2001). *The craft of teaching adults.* Toronto: Irwin Publishing.
Barrows, H., & Tamblyn, R. (1980). *Problem-based learning.* New York: Springer Publishing.
Biggs, J. B. (1973). Content to process. *Australian Journal of Education, 3,* 225–238.
Bloom, B. S., Englehart, M. D., Furst, E. J., Hill, L. M., & Krathwohl, D. R. (1956). *A taxonomy of educational objectives: Handbook I. The cognitive domain.* New York: Longman, Green.
Boak, G. (1998). *A complete guide to learning contracts.* Aldershot, England: Gower Publishing.
Bordage, G. (1994). Elaborated knowledge: A key to successful diagnostic thinking. *Academic Medicine, 69,* 883–885.
Boud, D., & Feletti, G. (1999). *The challenge of problem-based learning* (2nd ed.). London: Kogan Page.

Brookfield, S. (1990). *Understanding and facilitating adult learning.* San Francisco: Jossey-Bass.

Bruner, J. S. (1960). *The process of education.* Cambridge, MA: Harvard University Press.

Bruner, J. S. (1968). Act of discovery. In W. F. Romey (Ed.), *Inquiry techniques for teaching science.* Englewood Cliffs, NJ: Prentice Hall.

Dewey, J. (1938). *Experience and education.* New York: Collier Books.

Evans, M. (2001). Creating knowledge management skills in primary care residents. *ACP Journal Club,* September/October, A11–12.

Fabb, W. E., Heffernan, M. W., Phillips, W. A., & Stone, V. (1976). *Focus on learning in family practice.* Melbourne: Royal Australian College of General Practitioners.

Joyce, B., & Weil, M. (1992). *Models of teaching* (4th ed.). Boston: Allyn and Bacon.

Knowles, M. (1975). *Self-directed learning: A guide for learners and teachers.* Chicago: Follett Publishing.

Krathwohl, D. R., Bloom, B. S., & Masia, B. (1964). *A taxonomy of educational objectives: Handbook II. The affective domain.* New York: David Mackay.

MacKeracher, D. (1996). *Making sense of adult learning.* Toronto: Culture Concepts, Inc.

Mackway-Jones, K., & Walker, M. (1999). *Pocket guide to teaching for medical instructors.* London: BMJ Books.

Mager, R. F. (1962). *Preparing instructional objectives.* Belmont, CA: Fearon.

McLuhan, M. (1964). *Understanding media: The extension of man.* New York: McGraw-Hill.

McLuhan, M. (1967). *The medium is the message.* New York: Bantam.

Miller, G. E. (1962). *Teaching and learning in medical school.* Cambridge, MA: Harvard University Press.

Postman, N., & Weingartner, C. (1969). *Teaching as a subversive activity.* New York: Penguin Education.

Rogers, C. (1983). *Freedom to learn for the 80's.* New York: Merrill.

Schatz, I. (1993). Changes in undergraduate medical education. *Archives of Internal Medicine, 153,* 1045–1052.

Schon, D. (1987). *Educating the reflective practitioner.* San Francisco: Jossey-Bass.

Schwartz, S., & Bone, M. (1995). *Retelling, relating, reflecting.* Toronto: Irwin Publishing.

Shapiro, J., & Talbot, Y. (1991). Applying the concept of the reflective practitioner to understanding and teaching family medicine. *Family Medicine, 23,* 450–456.

Smith, C., & Irby, D. (1997). The roles of experience and reflection in ambulatory care education. *Academic Medicine, 72,* 32–35.

Tough, A. (1971). *The adult's learning projects.* Toronto: Ontario Institute for Studies in Education.

Westberg, J., & Jason, H. (1994). Fostering learners' reflection and self-assessment. *Family Medicine, 26,* 278–282.

Whitman, N., & Magill, M. (2000). The teaching moment. In P. Paulman, J. Susman, & C. Abboud (Eds.), *Precepting medical students in the office.* Baltimore: The Johns Hopkins University Press.

—2—

Teaching Skills in Ambulatory Care

After completing his reading on theories of learning, Dr. Z. Z. Smith thought that he needed to know more about teaching skills. He realized that there was a certain way he tended to teach when he had students in the practice. He also recognized that somehow he had learned this style of teaching; he knew it was not a birthright.

After thinking about it, his conclusion was that he had borrowed the style of his favorite teacher in medical school. It was the style he knew best and with which he was most comfortable. It seemed useful for the amount of time available in the office. His colleagues, however, used diverse teaching skills that differed greatly from his. It seemed possible to learn different styles for different situations. He challenged himself to learn more about teaching skills so that he could make explicit what style he was using most of the time and then adapt new ones to appropriate situations. Here is what he learned from several teaching skills workshops and from his reading of textbooks on this topic.

TEACHING STEPS

At every learning encounter, the teacher makes two important decisions even before getting to the teaching point. Often these are made without thinking and are just an instinctual response. The first is to choose a learner or teacher premise. The second is to choose a specific teaching skill to use in that circumstance. By understanding these first two steps, you can analyze what you usually do when you teach and then look at

15

some of the options available. You can then choose the best approach to optimize learning for that learner in a given situation. Your traditional, favorite approach is not necessarily the ideal way to enhance learning in every case.

Step 1

At a teaching encounter, you must choose one of two premises.

Choice One: Using the *learner premise*, you listen to case presentations from trainees or observe them directly with a patient. Based on what you have heard or seen, you organize and analyze the information about the trainees' knowledge and skills. You then use the outcome of this analysis in combination with your knowledge of the trainees' learning objectives as a basis for choosing a topic for the teaching encounter or for providing details to trainees on their performance.

Examples: The following are examples of the learner premise.

   1.   The student in your office for a gastrointestinal clinic presents the patient's history. Realizing that the student does not know the important risk factors for gallbladder disease, you discuss this topic with the entire group after seeing all the patients.
   2.   You observe a resident talking to a family about complications of proposed surgery, speaking quickly, using complex medical terms, and not allowing any time for questions. Later, you talk to the resident about what you observed and teach skills in talking to patients.
   3.   You assist a resident in inserting an intrauterine device. You observe that he fails to check the uterine position before beginning and has trouble with insertion of the sound. You teach him these two specific points by demonstrating them.

Choice Two: Using the *teacher premise*, you listen to a case presentation from a trainee. Based on the topic of the case, without making judgments on the knowledge or performance of that specific learner, you choose the topic on which to teach based on practice experience and previous encounters with trainees at that level of training.

Examples: The following are examples of the teacher premise.

1.   The fourth-year student presents a history of a patient with a peptic ulcer. You know that most students at that stage do not know much about ulcer treatment, so you proceed to review that topic with the student.

2.   A resident reports to you about several patients she has seen at the preoperative clinic. You ask the resident to sit in with you during the next patient meeting to observe your skills in telling patients about their proposed surgery.

3.   An intern tells you there is a patient with a seborrheic keratosis that she would like to remove. You tell her to watch you perform the procedure to see how you do it.

If you choose to operate from a learner premise, you are beginning to apply the principles of adult learning (e.g., teaching about learners' particular needs and letting them know how they are progressing). When choosing a teacher premise, you are using reception learning as your model, in which the teacher chooses a topic relevant to the clinical situation, often relying on his previous experience with trainees in these situations.

The skilled teacher will deliberately choose one of these premises to make the best of the learning encounter. Use a learner premise with more advanced trainees, who already possess considerable knowledge and experience and need to build on that. It is best suited for confident learners who want to hear about their performance.

Use the teacher premise with the novice or more anxious learner. In addition, this premise is appropriate when time is short and expediency will help get you back on schedule.

Step 2

At this point, teachers choose one of three fundamental teaching modes.

1.   *Telling:* Explicit statements to make a teaching point. It is the act of giving information or directing actions.

2.   *Asking:* Some form of questioning to make a teaching point.

3.   *Showing:* Illustrations or explanations in an orderly and detailed way of the essentials of the topic to be learned.

In many situations, you will find yourself switching from one mode to another. For example, you may begin by asking but then shift to a telling

mode because of time considerations, lack of knowledge on the part of
the learner, or questions from the learner. In addition, one mode may be
more effective in response to some situations than others, particularly if
you have chosen one premise over the other.

Table 2.1 lists specific teaching skills within each mode. Each mode
includes examples of when and under what conditions to use each skill.

TELLING

Directive Teaching

For use in learner premise situations, directive teaching is a most helpful
skill to master. Three ways of being directive are through the following
means:

1. *Description:* You can make a teaching point by describing in some
detail to the student her cognitive, affective, or motor performance. It
relates back to the trainee what he or she did and leads to a discussion
of how to correct the situation. An example is: "When discussing that
plan of investigation, you suggested two investigations, an abdominal
ultrasound and a liver-spleen scan. Any comments on your overall plan?"
(as opposed to saying "you are really overinvestigating that patient").

When using description, try to keep your statements

- Value free (not "that patient hated you," but "I noticed that patient
  was reluctant to answer your questions")
- Specific (not "you did not do a very good job on that cyst excision,"
  but "I saw these particular maneuvers with that surgery")

TABLE 2.1   Teaching Skills

Telling	Asking	Showing
Directive teaching	Socratic questioning	Demonstration
Comparison	Inquiry	Role modeling
Approval or reproach	Readiness	
Confrontation		
Response		

- Well timed (not "you remember that patient last week," but "let me tell you about your treatment plan for this last patient")
- Brief and manageable (not "here are the 10 problems with that history," but "let me tell you about two points concerning that history of knee pain") (Kaprelian & Gradeson, 1998).

By using description, you present a nonjudgmental set of facts to trainees on which to begin your teaching encounter and help trainees discover the points to be learned (i.e., a good example of discovery learning). It is particularly useful for trainees who react defensively to criticism when you present a predetermined conclusion to them that you have formulated from your observations. You may also use it with a learner who lacks confidence and who would become more anxious after hearing your conclusions and thus have difficulty making use of the information in that learning situation.

It is just as important to provide learners with descriptions of behavior, management plans, or procedures that are performed well or correctly (Neber, Gordon, Meyer, & Stevens, 1992). If learners are not provided with a mirror, they create their own images of how they are doing from incomplete or inaccurate clues. Some appropriate actions are pure luck; others are more deliberate. The learner does not actually know if she has done well. To become firmly established, competencies must be repeatedly rewarded in some fashion (O'Donohue & Ferguson, 2001). Reinforce the correct behavior, which is then learned and remembered. It is helpful to say "well done" but even more helpful to say "well done because. . . . "

2. *Metaphor:* Some teachers use metaphors to color the interaction between them and their trainees. An example is: "You were steamrolling that patient at the end of the interview." You might choose to use a metaphor with trainees who are having trouble grasping your point or who seem to learn best from visual images.

3. *Labeling:* The teacher can label an undesirable behavior, rather than providing a value-free description of it (an example of reception learning). For instance, you could tell a trainee that his recent actions were irresponsible instead of telling him about the behaviors that earned the "irresponsible" label (e.g., "Last night, you could not be reached on two occasions, you missed scrubbing in on the operating room case, and that blood sugar test never was done"). Because no trainee wants to be seen as irresponsible, the trainee may attend to what the teacher says after such a comment.

The risk with this method is that the trainee will turn off to learning once being struck by the label (e.g., "You were irresponsible"). The trainee focuses on the thought that he was irresponsible rather than learning from the circumstance. If this happens, ask the trainee about his reaction to your comment and then explore the behaviors that led to the labeling. The following exchange illustrates this point:

Teacher: "You have changed topics completely. Are you upset by my calling you irresponsible?"
Trainee: "I certainly am. It is very unfair."
Teacher: "Let's talk about what happened last night."

Use this teaching method when time is short or you want to emphasize a point. It works best with a mature learner. Avoid this strategy, however, with the learner who lacks self-confidence (Tiberius, 1995).

Comparison

Teachers can raise a learner's awareness of a shortcoming by comparing the learner's performance against an external authority such as a journal or textbook. The following exchange illustrates this point:

Learner: "It was impossible to get a history from this patient. He was all over the place and would not give me specific answers."
Teacher: "I also find these kinds of patients troubling. But a recent article in the *Journal of [Your Specialty]* provided some particularly good tips, such as . . ."

This is an effective and nonthreatening way to teach most trainees. According to the principles of adult learning (Knowles, 1980), learners thrive on, and learning is improved by, a nonthreatening, collegial environment. In medical settings, the physician teacher is automatically an authority figure to the learner. This hierarchy can create anxiety and interfere with learning. You establish a collegial atmosphere by transferring the authority from yourself to a book or journal. In addition, statements like "I also find these kinds of patients troubling" put learners at ease by helping them realize that you, too, have similar learning concerns. Learning is now collegial, and you have created an adult learning environment. Comparison is especially useful for learners new to your office or for those who seem anxious in one-on-one learning situations.

Approval or Reproach

You may choose to make strong statements of approval or reproach to describe a learner's behavior. With such a statement, you rapidly emphasize the behavior you wish to highlight. Such a strong declaration immediately draws the learner's thoughts to the issue. Use this method when time is short and you want to bring a learning point to the student's attention in a brief encounter. For example, "You were entirely undependable during that labor and delivery last night," or "You demonstrated a tremendous sense of responsibility when you were readily available to manage that high-risk labor and delivery last night."

All learners appreciate the praise inherent in an approval statement. Use statements of reproach sparingly, or they will lose meaning to the learner. With new or self-conscious trainees, statements of reproach may evoke feelings of insecurity or defensiveness and thus have little effect.

Confrontation

Confrontation is often frowned on in teaching because it may be interpreted by the trainee as a put-down and actually block any chance for learning by shutting off the trainee's willingness to learn. In some instances, when you have tried other techniques previously and the trainee does not seem to be getting the point, a direct, forceful statement may bring the issue to the trainee's attention. Here is an example.

Trainee: "We cannot keep talking about this. I have other people waiting to see me."

Teacher: "John, you keep looking for ways to avoid this issue we are trying to discuss. It is making me very angry."
Or, "It seems to me that you want to avoid this situation. What do you think?"

The danger in using confrontation is that sometimes the students perceive the encounter as severely critical, and they may not be willing to hear it (Irby, 1986).

Response

In medical teaching, response is a commonly used method. In using a learner premise, the teacher recognizes a teaching point to be made and tells the learner in response to the specific circumstance. Alternatively, the learner may ask a question, and the teacher provides a straight answer. In responding, it is important to be brief and concise even though you have the urge to pass on as much information and detail as possible at one time. In the ambulatory setting, each case dredges up a deluge of facts and tips that could be told to the learner. In your response, choose to include points that are directly relevant to the learner's identified objectives. Remember the teachable moment. Base your response on what is immediately related to the patient encounter. Try to exclude items that may be attractive to you because of your own personal interests or only remotely connected to the case at hand (Fabb, Heffernan, Phillips, & Stone, 1976).

It is also the experience of some teachers that, having covered something previously with a learner, the next time the topic comes up it is as if you never discussed it previously. Unfortunately, students cannot learn as fast as teachers can speak. Research has shown that learners have difficulty remembering large bits of information and can only absorb and retain certain amounts at one given sitting. Remember to limit the bits of information provided to the student, realizing that the learner will have other opportunities to learn a given point and that you do not have to cover everything.

At the end of your response, to help ensure that your points were clearly understood and to enhance retention, you can ask the learner the following:

"Did I confuse you at all?"

"Do you have any questions?"

"Did I cover too much?

"Is it all clear to you?"

"Can I repeat any of the points for you?"

Even if the learner requires no further response, these questions also provide a momentary break before the next teaching point or before returning to the patient (Quirk, 1994).

When responding, you may not be sure if the learners have grasped the material or become lost along the way. Here are three skills that help in these situations.

Checking Out: This approach helps you understand the emotional state of the trainee when you are aware that the trainee may have missed your point. You verbalize to the trainee your impression of her current state of mind and await a response.

Trainee: "That sounds like a good plan for treating this patient's symptoms. But I think he needs a barium enema before we use that treatment."

Teacher: "From this conversation, you seem to be quite anxious about this patient, and I think you may have missed my point about the need for an initial trial of therapy. Any particular reason for this anxiety?"

Trainee: "Yes. The last patient I had like this one, I missed a colon cancer."

Paraphrasing: In discussions with trainees, you may periodically cover a few points in succession and not be quite sure if the trainee has gotten the teaching points clearly. It is helpful then to stop and ask the trainee to paraphrase what you have been saying. Ask the trainee to reword or restate the information in a shortened manner to see if the teaching point is clearly understood. For example, "I have covered a lot of points in the last few minutes. It might be helpful if you could restate some of them in your own words, so that we could clear up any confusing points."

Summarizing: After discussing a few learning points with learners, it is helpful to summarize them as you conclude or before you go on to another point. This technique helps learners to extract the important points from what may have been a lengthy conversation. To summarize, simply list the teaching points in a clear, concise manner, covering the essential points of the exchange and trying to relate them to the learner's objectives. For example, "The three points we covered about proteinuria are: get a fresh morning specimen, do a microscopic assessment, and then order the 24-hour urine test for total protein."

There is an added benefit to this technique. If the summary is not a faithful reflection of the conversation from the learners' viewpoint, they will raise this issue and alert you to some misunderstanding of the teaching point.

ASKING

Socratic Questioning

When choosing the asking mode, you may wish to use an indirect manner of questioning. This is a particularly good example of discovery learning, in which learners are guided to the information. Mature adult learners thrive on this approach. Known as Socratic questioning, a series of questions is provided to learners to gradually increase their own awareness of the teaching point. The questions are usually sequenced, from general issues to the specific.

This method is more than just asking questions. It is asking questions to encourage independent thinking. It helps learners see the logical connection from point to point. The questions help learners explore what knowledge they already possess and how to apply it to novel situations (Ende, Pomerantz, & Erickson, 1995).

Examples: The following are examples of this method.

1.   *Learner premise:* A student has just seen a case, and it is clear from her presentation that she is unsure of the differential diagnosis of abdominal pain in a 24-year-old woman. You think that you should discuss this topic with her. Some possible questions to ask, in sequence, include the following:

"What do you think is this patient's major problem?"

"Where would you start in dealing with this abdominal pain?"

"What do you already know about abdominal pain?"

"What else might help you think of the causes of abdominal pain?"

"How might you differentiate the causes of abdominal pain?"

"What features of the history in this case help you to pinpoint the diagnosis?"

2.   *Teacher premise:* A resident works in your office every Friday morning. The next patient has been referred because of chronic headaches. Some possible questions to ask include the following:

"The next case is one referred for headaches. What are the causes of chronic headaches?"

"How might you better group the causes?"

"What will help you pinpoint the specific cause?"

"How do questions about the time course help you distinguish the different kinds of headaches?"

Avoid a guessing game with the resident. Because you have a teaching point in mind as you phrase the questions, you may inadvertently lead the resident to a very specific point. The resident will pick up on this and try to guess the answers for which you are unconsciously probing.

Use the Socratic technique when there is enough time to allow for a series of questions and their responses, such as at lunch, at the end of the day during a chart review, or perhaps during a canceled appointment. Avoid the technique with anxious learners who have a poor knowledge base, for each succeeding question will just raise more panic. It is best for learners who have considerable information on hand and just need guidance to organize what they already know.

Inquiry

This method is probably the most common one used by doctors in medical teaching. Although this term has a somewhat negative connotation, inquiry just means the use of a series of questions, usually flowing from the response to the previous one.

The purpose of inquiry is to test what the learner knows and then fill in the gaps. You can also find out about the learner's thinking processes and decision making by direct inquiry. Use it when time is short, but asking is preferred to telling or showing (Benzie, 1998).

Because you are finding out what learners know, you can use this information as part of their evaluation. Based on students' learning objectives, you can also let them know how they are progressing. Remember that every time you ask a series of questions, you automatically evaluate students' knowledge by the accuracy and depth of their responses. Let them know what you think. For example, you might say, "That's excellent. You have a clear and detailed understanding of the treatment of glaucoma."

Another possible comment is the following: "As part of your objectives this month, you were going to learn about the laboratory tests for lupus. You seem to have accomplished that. As we discussed this last patient, you were able to tell me exactly which tests to order in this circumstance and why."

Finally, if a student is having difficulty, you might say, "You are having difficulty answering any questions about this patient's middle ear problem. Let's talk about where you might get some more information on this topic."

Inquiry differs from Socratic questioning in that the questions are very specific from the beginning rather than general, and exact answers are expected. In addition, Socratic questioning explores the thinking of the learner. With inquiry, the learner is required to come up with the answer that you already have in mind.

The skilled user of inquiry will avoid the authoritarian, emphatic series of questions that can intimidate or even freeze the learner. The questions can be presented in a collegial manner with encouragement as the answer is provided by the learner. Say that it is acceptable to be wrong, to venture guesses and opinions as part of learning (Schwenk & Whitman, 1993).

With inquiry use questions that are the following:

- Clear
- Brief (one question at a time)
- Single focus
- Divergent (allow more than one acceptable answer and broad thinking)
- Open-ended (short answers are insufficient) (Mackway-Jones & Walker, 1999).

You can also ask questions to challenge the resident at different levels of thinking (Bloom, 1956). The simplest, lower-level question elicits a yes/ no answer to a list of facts. A higher level question involves asking the resident to apply their knowledge in a novel way. At the highest level, questions will require analysis or synthesis, i.e., breaking down knowledge into its components and reformulating the trainee's thinking.

For example:

"Is this a classic type migraine headache? (yes/no question)

"What are the possible causes of this patient's headache?" (remembering facts)

"Explain how sumatriptan works to relieve migraine headache? (application of knowledge)

Compare the clinical features of migraine and tension headache? (analysis)

"Using evidence based medicine, defend your choice for management of acute migraine headache?" (synthesis)

You can be even more helpful with inquiry by assisting learners in delving into their memory. Learners probably have most of the information stored in their memory and simply need help to access it (Elstein, Shulman, & Sprafka, 1978). Adult learners thrive on searching for and discovering learning material for themselves. Some learners cannot think of the answer when first asked but say "oh, yes" with a nodding head when the answer becomes apparent. The theory is that most learners possess abundant knowledge, but it is stored and accessed in a particular way for each student. Research has shown that when learners do not come up with the correct answer, it is not usually because they do not have the knowledge. It is because the knowledge is stored in their memories in a way that they cannot get at it (Bordage, Grant, & Marsden, 1990). Increasing experience is accompanied by increasing accessibility of the knowledge stored in memory. With increasing practice, discussion, and thought, the doctor will gradually alter the shape of memorized knowledge until it becomes finely tuned to the needs of clinical practice, generalizable from case to case, and accessible when it is needed (Gruppen, 1997).

To use this strategy, affirm with learners at the outset that they have the knowledge to find the diagnosis, plan the management, and so on. Then direct your questions to get at learners' stored memory. Research shows that it is better to guide the learner through this process, promoting reflection, than to directly tell him the answers (Taylor, Dunn, & Lipsky, 1993).

- Prod the student's memory by reviewing particular points of the history and physical examination.
- Relate this case to previous ones.
- Discuss one issue at a time.
- Break down each issue, idea, or concept to a less demanding level.
- Ask the student to combine pieces of information.
- Rephrase your question in different words. Try a "what if" question (What if the patient were 30 years old instead of 50?).
- Review the previous points by going back over what has just been discussed to attempt to arouse memory.
- Prompt the student with simple words or statements that will act as clues to stored memory.
- Summarize the process that brought the student to the answer, right or wrong.

Readiness

When beginning to ask questions, be prepared to deal with blocks in students' ability to deal with questions. These obstructions must be cleared up before students are ready to move on (Guilbert, 1981). For example, you might say, "Let's stop for a minute and discuss what seems to be upsetting you so much. I remember that patient who died when you were first on call. That death upset me. I was wondering if this is what's upsetting you?"

Another problem of readiness is a mismatch between the developmental level of the student and the message being communicated. The student may have to become more sophisticated in that area before being able to understand the message. For example, a third-year medical student in your office on an elective would have difficulty understanding the ethical choices in the investigation of an Alzheimer's patient with anemia because of a lack of knowledge of the differential diagnosis and natural history of the disease.

SHOWING

Demonstration

It is common in ambulatory care teaching to demonstrate to trainees motor skills and even some affective skills (Whitman & Schwenk, 1997). Demonstration is the illustration or explanation of various procedural or technical skills in an orderly and detailed way. When demonstrating a new skill to a trainee (Foley & Smilansky, 1980), you should:

1.   Find what the trainee may already know about the procedure and work from that starting point. There is no use in wasting time on what the trainee already knows and can do.
2.   Review the procedure with a diagram or verbally before actually beginning it on the patient. Break it down into its component parts, each of which is easily digestible.
3.   Give a running commentary of what you are doing as you proceed.
4.   Comment on the variety of approaches for a given situation.
5.   Be clear, concise, and brief in your explanation.
6.   Review the procedure with the trainee after you have completed it, and allow for any questions.
7.   Reserve time for the most difficult parts.

In ambulatory care settings, you will often be seeing patients simultaneously with trainees. Remember to call trainees to your office to examine a patient who demonstrates any special clinical findings that trainees might not otherwise experience or those that relate to trainees' learning objectives.

Demonstration may also be used effectively for teaching about the medical record. Illustrate for your trainees:

- Well-organized patient charts, with a problem list, flow charts of laboratory tests, etc.
- Concise, legible, and accurate documentation of an office visit
- Helpful referral note to a consulting physician
- Comprehensive consultation letter to the referring physician

Even demonstrate to learners your reasoning in the midst of case decision making. Think out loud. Be reflective and articulate about your thinking process. This allows learners to see how skilled, experienced doctors approach a clinical problem (Irby, 1995).

Role Modeling

Role modeling can be defined as facilitating learning by personally being the example of the attitude or concept to be learned. Role models are persons whose behaviors, personal styles, and specific attributes are emulated by others (Ricer, 2000). We act as role models for our trainees all the time, whether we like it or not, or whether we are aware of it or not. They constantly observe what we do and say, and they integrate lessons to be learned from these actions (Wright & Carrese, 2002). These learned behaviors can be both positive and negative ones. Role modeling is a powerful learning tool, for trainees quickly pick up the codes of conduct of the physician and act accordingly (Irby, 1986).

Be aware that your interactions and attitudes influence students. Teachers who perceive themselves as role models and make use of that role are more highly rated by learners (Wright, Kern, Kolodner, Howard, & Brancati, 1998). Use role modeling as an effective teaching tool by consciously and deliberately modeling behavior in areas where learning needs to be enhanced. For example, in a second-year course on interviewing, students were able to observe "charismatic role models" taking a history (Siegler, Reaven, Lipinski, & Stocking, 1987). This intervention improved scores of students' attitudes about interpersonal skills as well as the doctor-patient relationship.

Ambulatory teachers in medicine can promote learning through role modeling in the following:

- Time management
- Intellectual curiosity
- Continuing self-education
- Critical analysis of information
- Sensitivity, respect, and compassion for patients (Hekelman & Blasé, 1996)
- Cooperation and mutual respect among specialties
- Collaboration with other disciplines and respect for the specific knowledge and skills that other health professionals have (Prideaux et al., 2000)
- Interest in professional associations, community advocacy, and non-medical lifestyle activities
- Balance of professional, personal, and family responsibilities (Ficklin, Browne, Powell, & Carter, 1988)

Role modeling is particularly helpful for novice students who have little experience and knowledge on which to base their learning. Or, it may be used when a student or resident first comes to the office and you ask her to follow you to assist in her initiation to the clinical environment (Wilkerson & Sarkin, 1998). It is especially useful when teaching on affective topics such as patient interviewing, health counseling, or obtaining consent for surgery. For example, suppose that a student is having difficulty taking a history from a patient. You could say, "Let's go and interview this patient together. Watch me and focus on how I get the patient to give more specific details on the characteristics of the pain. Then we will review these points afterward." Conversely, more experienced students might be happier if you just highlight some areas for improvement and then let them go and do it.

REFERENCES

Benzie, D. (1998). Levels of questioning for learners. *Family Medicine, 30,* 12–13.

Bloom, B. S., Englehart, M. A., Furst, E. J., Hill, L. M., & Krathwohl, D. R. (1956). *A taxonomy of educational objectives: Handbook I. The cognitive domain.* New York: Longman, Green.

Bordage, G., Grant, J., & Marsden, P. (1990). Quantitative assessment of diagnostic ability. *Medical Education, 24,* 413–425.

Elstein, A., Shulman, L., & Sprafka, S. (1978). *Medical problem solving: An analysis of clinical reasoning.* Cambridge, MA: Harvard University Press.

Ende, J., Pomerantz, A., & Erickson, F. (1995). Preceptors' strategies for correcting residents in an ambulatory care medicine setting: A qualitative analysis. *Academic Medicine, 70,* 224–227.

Fabb, W. E., Heffernan, M. W., Phillips, W. A., & Stone, V. (1976). *Focus on learning in family practice.* Melbourne: Royal Australian College of General Practitioners.

Ficklin, F., Browne, V., Powell, R., & Carter, J. (1988). Faculty and house staff members as role models. *Journal of Medical Education, 63,* 392–396.

Foley, R., & Smilansky, J. (1980). *Teaching techniques: A handbook for health professionals.* New York: McGraw-Hill.

Gruppen, L. (1997). Implications of cognitive research for ambulatory care education. *Academic Medicine, 72,* 117–120.

Guilbert, J. (1981). *Educational handbook for health personnel* (Offset Publication No. 35). Geneva: World Health Organization.

Hekelman, F., & Blasé, J. (1996). Excellence in clinical teaching: The core of the mission. *Academic Medicine, 71,* 738–742.

Irby, D. (1986). Clinical teaching and the clinical teacher. *Medical Education, 61,* 35–45.

Irby, D. (1995). Teaching and learning in ambulatory settings: A thematic review of the literature. *Academic Medicine, 70,* 898–931.

Kaprelian, V., & Gradeson, M. (1998). Effective use of feedback. *Family Medicine, 30,* 406–407.

Knowles, M. (1980). *Modern practice of adult education.* Chicago: Follett Publishing.

Mackway-Jones, K., & Walker, M. (1999). *Pocket guide to teaching for medical instructors.* London: BMJ Books.

Neber, J., Gordon, K., Meyer, B., & Stevens, N. (1992). A five-step microskills model of clinical teaching. *Journal of the American Board of Family Practice, 5,* 419–424.

O'Donohue, W., & Ferguson, K. (2001). *The psychology of B. F. Skinner.* San Francisco: Sage Publications.

Prideaux, D., Alexander, H., Bower, A., Dacre, J., Haist, S., Jolly, B., Norcini, J., Roberts, T., Rothman, A., Rowe, R., & Tallett, S. (2000). Clinical teaching: Maintaining an educational role for doctors in the new health care environment. *Medical Education, 34,* 820–826.

Quirk, M. (1994). *How to learn and teach in medical school: A learner-centered approach.* Springfield, IL: Charles C. Thomas.

Ricer, R. (2000). In P. Paulman, J. Susman, & C. Abboud (Eds.), *Precepting medical students in the office.* Baltimore: Johns Hopkins University Press.

Schwenk, T., & Whitman, N. (1993). *Residents as teachers: A guide to educational practice.* Salt Lake City: University of Utah School of Medicine.

Siegler, M., Reaven, N., Lipinski, R., & Stocking, C. (1987). Effect of role model clinicians on students' attitudes in a second year course on introduction to the patient. *Journal of Medical Education, 62,* 935–937.

Taylor, C., Dunn, T., & Lipsky, M. (1993). Extent to which guided-discovery teaching strategies were used by 20 preceptors in family medicine. *Academic Medicine, 68,* 385–387.

Tiberius, R. (1995). *Small group teaching: A trouble-shooting guide.* Toronto: OISE Press.

Whitman, N., & Schwenk, K. (1997). *The physician as teacher.* Baltimore: Williams and Wilkins.

Wilkerson, L., & Sarkin, R. (1998). Teaching the teachers: Is it effective? *Academic Medicine, 73,* S67–S69.

Wright, S., Kern, D., Kolodner, K., Howard, D., & Brancati, F. (1998). Attributes of excellent attending-physician role models. *New England Journal of Medicine, 339,* 1986–1993.

Wright, S., & Carresa, J. (2002). Excellence in role modelling: Insight and perspectives from the pros. *Canadian Medical Association Journal, 167,* 638–642.

—3—

Setting Up the Office for Teaching

Several years after joining the multispecialty clinic, Dr. Z. Z. Smith became the director. He agreed with the local medical school to have senior medical students and residents come to the clinic for their ambulatory training. He thinks back about the meeting he had with his colleagues after being approached by the associate dean of the medical school about the idea of using the clinic for ambulatory teaching. He recalls that, at first, most were against it. They made the following comments:

> "We already teach at the hospital. Why do we have to do more teaching in the office as well?"

> "We never had ambulatory experience when we were training, and we seem to be quite capable doctors. The students do not get enough hospital experience as it is, with all those electives and seminar time."

> "The residents will just get in the way. Can you imagine how much they will slow us down?"

> "Where will we find enough patients for our clinic groups?"

> "It will cost us a fortune to have the students here."

> "We really do not have any extra rooms for them to see patients."

> "Our patients do not want to see students. They come here to see us as their doctors."

Other colleagues, however, supported the idea at once. They said the following:

"Ambulatory medical teaching is the future of medical education."

"We are all committed to medical teaching and enjoy it. We just need to reorient our thinking to the ambulatory setting, just as we have reoriented our thinking for patient care from the hospital to the outpatient setting. Can you imagine 15 years ago trying to implement the plans for outpatient investigations and treatments we now take for granted?"

"It really should not cost us that much or anything at all. The residents may even make us more efficient and produce some extra income to make up for any shortfall."

"I think there are more empty rooms at certain times of the day than we think there are."

"You know how much our patients are impressed by our teaching credentials. And many of them really enjoy talking to students and feel good about helping them in their education."

By the end of the meeting, those in favor of ambulatory teaching carried the day. Dr. Smith was charged with the responsibility of organizing the details and reporting back to the group for final approval.

WHERE WILL THEY WORK?

The next morning Dr. Smith came into the office early before any patients had arrived. He looked around the waiting room and the reception desk, and peered into some of the examining rooms. He was frozen by a brief surge of panic. His colleagues were right. Where will residents work? How will a medical school clinic group fit into this office space?

He slumped into his chair and pondered the problem. Soon it struck him that at least a third of the physicians in the group do not come to the office in the morning. Some are in the operating room. Others work at the hospital in the morning or afternoon doing procedures. Dr. Smith decided to ask the office manager to draw up a schedule of exactly when each office and examining room is occupied. The following are our recommended steps.

Preparation of Your Office for Teaching

1. Draw up an office plan or list of all available rooms. Note when they are occupied or available. This will give you an idea of how many trainees you can accommodate and at what times.

2. Try to create blocks of examining rooms that can be used when a student is in the office, for students or residents need to be near the physician with whom they are working. Remember that the more junior students need more time to see a patient. Have other rooms available where the teaching physician can continue to see patients at the same time.

3. Consider converting one room into an area where trainees may be observed unobtrusively. There are several inexpensive ways to approach this:

   a. The least expensive is to purchase a tape recorder and have it sit on the desk where the student is interviewing patients. The student can turn it on for particular patients or have it running for the entire session.

   b. You can prepare a room for direct observation by mounting a video camera with a wide-angle lens in one corner. (The same camera that stores use for detecting shoplifters is small, inexpensive, and ready for mounting on a simple bracket.) The wire can then be led to almost any room above the ceiling tiles, where it is attached to a standard videocassette recorder and a television set. (You might use the office coffee room for this.) The entire equipment can be purchased for a $1,000 or even less. Most medical schools have funds for such a purchase, and it could be made part of the arrangement with the associate dean.

   c. Although supplanted by more inexpensive video equipment, a one-way mirror can be built into any wall for about $500.

4. Make trainees (especially senior ones) feel part of the office, particularly if they are to be there for an extended period. Print some personalized business cards and prescription pads for them. Provide an individual mailbox and telephone message slot, similar to the other physicians. In addition, consider adding their names to the list of physicians on your office wall using a sign that can be easily changed. These maneuvers help patients integrate these physicians as part of your practice and help with issues of continuity of care.

5. Remember to make use of other resources in the community (Richards, 1996). There may not be room in your clinic each day for trainees. This creates an opportunity for trainees to learn about the role of other organizations and health professionals in the community. With little firsthand knowledge about the community, the trainee has only his own life experiences to draw on when assessing patients' overall needs. Expand that viewpoint by arranging for trainees to visit (depending on your specialty):

- Public health units
- Home care organizations (do home visits)
- Community mental health services, including those serving specific cultural groups
- Assisted-living facilities or nursing homes
- Hospice care
- Family-planning clinics
- Local pharmacy
- Home health services—assistive devices, oxygen supply

WHAT WILL THE PATIENTS THINK?

As he was finishing his examination of Mr. Jones that day, the patient said to Dr. Smith, "Thank you so much for helping me with this illness. It's been so beneficial to have you there throughout. I could not have made it without you." Because teaching had been on his mind all day, his first reaction was "Could Mr. Jones have handled a student being involved in his care?" Would patients leave the practice if they started to have students coming to the office?

Preparation of the Patients for Teaching

In our experience, many patients look on the teaching aspect of a practice in a positive manner. Patients are, in general, receptive to students and residents, who they believe increase the attention given to the patient (Hajioff & Birchall, 1999). It is unusual for patients to leave a practice or refuse to attend one solely because there may be trainees involved in their care. Teaching actually gives a high profile to the practice and, in many circumstances, increases patient satisfaction (Deutsch, 1997; Grayson, Klein, Lugo, & Visintainer, 1998; Simon, Peters, Christiansen, & Fletcher,

2000). You do not see patients avoid teaching hospitals for fear of trainee involvement! The challenge is to prepare patients properly to help them understand the role of a teaching practice and the role of the student in their care.

1. The practice as a teaching unit and its link to the university can be proudly emphasized. The medical school or specialty department should present each teaching practice with an impressive-looking plaque to hang in the waiting room, near the front entrance doorway, or next to the list of doctors. See Figure 3.1 for an example.
2. As each new patient registers, many practices give a brochure that

UNIVERSITY OF MAIN STREET

DR. Z.Z. SMITH

is participating with the University of Main Street in the training of doctors. You may be asked to be attended by a trainee under the supervision of your physician. Your cooperation is much appreciated.

Jon Doe, M.D.
Dean

FIGURE 3.1 Sample plaque indicating practice as teaching unit and its link to the university.

Welcome to the Clinics of Main Street. In this unit, the doctors and nurses provide care for patients of all ages involving many branches of medical care. In addition, there is access to all departments and services of the Main Street Hospital.

The clinic is affiliated with the University of Main Street. We are involved with teaching new doctors and student doctors from the medical school. For this reason, on some of your visits, you may see a medical student or doctor in training in one of the specialties. Your own physician will always be directly involved in your care.

In some circumstances, to assist in our teaching, your visit may be recorded on videotape for review with the trainee and your physician. If you would prefer not to be involved in this teaching program, please notify us. This will in no way diminish the quality of care you receive at the Clinics of Main Street.

FIGURE 3.2   Sample brochure summarizing teaching activities.

outlines the routines of the office. Included in that brochure should be a summary of the teaching activities of the practice. Figure 3.2 is a sample of what might be included to inform patients of the doctors' teaching role.

3. Some practices establish a volunteer registry of patients who are particularly interested in helping out with the teaching programs. This is more important if your practice becomes involved with early medical school teaching of clinical methods, interviewing skills, or other medical or surgical activities that require a prolonged period with each patient. Two groups of patients may be especially interested in this type of involvement:

    a. Older patients or isolated individuals who appreciate the opportunity to get out and talk with young people.

    b. Those who recognize the importance of medical education and respond to the chance of being involved in this role. To some, it is as important as any other volunteer community service.

    A special handout can be prepared for distribution or a poster put up in the waiting room to advertise the need for volunteers. See Figures 3.3 and 3.4 for some examples.

4. When patients call for appointments, most practices find it beneficial to inform them in advance that a student or resident will be involved in their care. There are, of course, different circumstances depending on the level of the student's training.

    a. For undergraduate students, who usually work with the doctor, tell patients when they call for an appointment that the doctor has a student from the medical school working with her that day. The patient may be seen first by the student, but the doctor will also see the patient directly.

THE CLINICS OF MAIN STREET

This office requires volunteers to assist with teaching interviewing skills to medical students from the University of Main Street.

What is required?
Approximately 2 hours. Appointment times would usually be Tuesday afternoons.

What would you do?
Be interviewed by a medical student about your health history.

If interested, please see the receptionist for details.

FIGURE 3.3   Sample poster advertising the need for volunteers.

b. For more senior trainees, who work independently, appointments can be booked specifically for that trainee with the level of training and teaching role explained more fully at the office.

Some patients are reluctant to be involved with trainees. Schedule appointments with them on another day when students are not present.

❦

VOLUNTEERS REQUIRED FOR TEACHING

Are you interested in helping medical students to develop their interviewing skills?

Physicians at the Clinics of Main Street are teaching interviewing skills to first year medical students. The course introduces students to the skills in conducting a good interview. We require the assistance of people who would be willing to be interviewed by several students about their medical problems.

The course is taught on Tuesday afternoons. If you are interested, and have an hour or two to volunteer, please fill out the information below. We would like to check with your personal physician prior to arranging a time for you to come.

Name: _____

Phone Number: _____

Your Doctor: _____

❦

FIGURE 3.4   Sample handout advertising the need for volunteers.

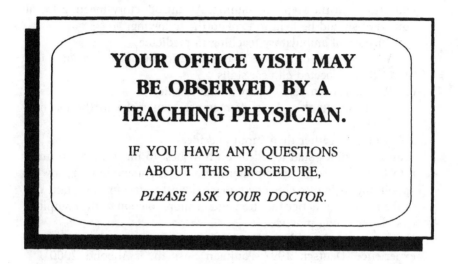

FIGURE 3.5   Sample sign indicating that direct observation is part of teaching practices.

It is the authors' experience that less than 10 percent of patients express reluctance to be involved with a trainee.

5. If direct observation is part of your teaching practice, carefully explain this in the information brochure and have a sign clearly visible in every room that informs patients. Figure 3.5 illustrates such a sign.

HOW WILL THE OFFICE STAFF COPE?

Dr. Smith had his weekly meeting with the office manager that afternoon. He approached the meeting with trepidation, and for good reason. First, he had to calm down the manager and then educate her about this new activity and its importance. After a while, he was able to persuade her that the presence of students would greatly enhance staff morale, add some more prestige to working at the office, and reduce turnover of the ancillary staff. The manager agreed to establish a plan to educate the office staff members in their new role.

Preparation of the Office Staff for Teaching

1. All staff must understand the role that the office plays as a teaching practice. Do not assume that clerical staff or nurses know about medical

education and the steps in training. An introductory meeting for all
your staff should be held to explain the following:
   a.   Purpose of ambulatory teaching in medicine
   b.   Various levels of trainees that will be in the office and some idea
        of their expected clinical skills
   c.   Role that trainees will play in the practice
   d.   Contribution that the staff members can make to the teaching
        program
   e.   A plan to gather their input and ideas
2. Canvas the office staff for ideas on how best to integrate the trainees
   into the office (e.g., appointment bookings, patient flow, follow-up
   appointments, etc.). This encourages them to play an important role
   in the teaching practice function and be more tolerant of the complexities of a teaching practice.
3. Here are examples of how the office staff can enhance the educational
   experience (Deutsch, 1997; Paulman, Susman, & Abboud, 2000).
   a.   *Medical secretaries:* They can help trainees learn proper dictation
        techniques, charting tips, and use of office electronic medical re-
        cords and can give advice on general office supplies and equipment
        (e.g., where to order supplies, what size stationery and envelopes,
        etc.). The secretaries can educate trainees about preparing referral
        letters used by primary care physicians or reply letters after consul-
        tation for specialty disciplines. They might highlight the need for a
        referral letter to indicate clearly the reason for referral, the patient's
        ongoing medical conditions and treatments, tests and results com-
        pleted to date, and the urgency of the consultation request (New-
        ton, Eccles, & Hutchinson, 1992). The consultant's reply letter
        needs to be prepared promptly and should not repeat detail already
        known about the patient's history and background. Referring doc-
        tors want information regarding diagnosis, clinical findings, test
        results, treatment options, expected outcomes including risks and
        benefits, and any psychosocial concerns (Tattersall et al., 1995).
   b.   *Receptionists:* They can demonstrate to trainees how to schedule
        appointments; arrange follow-up visits; cope with "walk-in" pa-
        tients; make referrals; book hospital beds, operating rooms, and
        laboratory tests; deal with difficult or demanding patients; and
        organize time during the daily schedule to respond to telephone
        calls.
   c.   *Nurses and nurse practitioners:* They play a broad role in the ambula-
        tory training experience. They may instruct trainees on performing
        office procedures (e.g., electrocardiogram or spirometry), manag-

ing common clinical problems, taking a concise history, using community resources, and maintaining patient flow. They can educate residents about telephone triage and how and what conditions can be safely managed over the telephone within your specialty. Role play is an effective method to simulate common telephone situations and allow trainees to practice talking through typical scenarios within your discipline (see chapter 4).

d. *Managers and administrators:* They can provide trainees, especially senior ones about to enter practice, with the details of setting up and running an office. The topics to emphasize could include office design, hiring and training staff, performance appraisal, medical records, accounting and bookkeeping, and dealing with insurance companies and third-party agencies.

4. The office staff have a critical role in integrating the trainees into the daily practice, especially in how the patients view the students. Make sure the staff understand that the students are to be treated as members of the team, not as interlopers or observers for a brief period. Here are a few suggestions.

a. The staff should direct telephone calls from patients to the trainee who saw the patient.

b. They should reaffirm with patients that the trainees, though temporary, are an integral part of the office.

c. Staff should even attempt to contact students regarding their patients on days when the student is away from the office, instead of asking one of the regular physicians.

WILL THE OTHER DOCTORS GET INVOLVED?

Dr. Smith sat down at the end of day to review his progress. So far, so good, he thought to himself. He was certain that the staff could manage with the existing physical space. The office staff seemed quite excited and had a plan to educate their patients. He was still concerned, however, that his colleagues were reluctant to climb aboard. After spending time with all this organizing, would they respond to the call? Dr. Smith realized that he had to have a carefully thought-out plan for the medical staff as well.

Preparation of the Physicians for Teaching

1. Allow some time for the idea of ambulatory care teaching to register. Most physicians who get involved with ambulatory care teaching have taught previously in a hospital. In general, they enjoy teaching. To

make the transition to ambulatory teaching, it is important to work out the organizational kinks so that the physicians will feel more comfortable about trainees being in the office. They need guidance on how to convert the lengthy hospital teaching sessions into targeted, highly selective, brief encounters. Convene a follow-up meeting to outline the completion of the plan for having students in the office. Allow time for comments and further suggestions to be received from the teaching physicians.

2. Some physicians wonder how their patients will react to the trainees. Some may resent the interference of a trainee. There should be opportunity to air these concerns at a meeting. Here is an example from the authors' practice that highlights this issue.

    In our office, there is an active obstetrical practice. Obstetrical training is an important part of our education program (Carroll, 1986). To ensure that trainees have an adequate patient load overall as well as appropriate supervision of their own patients, a policy was implemented whereby each obstetrical couple is assigned to a resident and teaching physician. The patient is seen on alternate visits by the resident or physician. This applies whether the patient was originally in the practice of the physician or entered the practice as a patient of a resident. At first, some physicians were resistant to the idea. Some comments were "Obstetrical patients like to have their own doctor," "Obstetrical patients are so nervous, they will never handle the two doctors," or "We will lose patients and get no referrals."

    The patients, however, never seemed to have a problem with the alternate visits plan and appreciated the time the residents spent talking to them. They also liked the fact that with two doctors it was much more likely that someone they knew well would be at their delivery. During the 20 years of this joint visit program, there have been no patients lost for refusal to participate, the obstetrical load originally doubled and has remained stable, and there are even more referrals from other physicians for obstetrical care as knowledge of the excellent academic program spreads.

3. Most physicians are unsure of how and what to teach in an ambulatory setting. They may be comfortable with the content within their specialty but need to adjust their teaching to the learning opportunities of ambulatory care. The focus of their teaching within their specialty can be organized with the following in mind:

    •   Prevalence of problems in the specialty seen in ambulatory setting versus hospital setting

- Investigation of specific presenting complaints of outpatients
- Treatment of common problems of the specialty in an ambulatory setting
- Focused history and physical examination
- Patient follow-up: timing, frequency of laboratory tests, and so on
- Procedures that can be done in the outpatient setting: investigation and treatment
- Writing consultation or referral letters
- Interaction with patients before firm diagnosis is established
- Preparation of patients for admission to hospital (i.e., preadmission testing, preoperative assessment)
- Use of community resources and agencies for prehospital and posthospital management (e.g., home care agencies, palliative care services, etc.)
- Telephone management
- Enhancement of patient compliance
- Interaction with families
- Time factor: diagnosis is sometimes made over time as disease develops
- Health maintenance and prevention
- Interaction with third-party agencies

4. Physicians have two fears as they begin to teach in the ambulatory care setting: loss of income and loss of referrals. Here is a helpful view of these issues.
   a. Adding trainees to your practice is probably income neutral. More senior trainees bring in extra income as they see additional patients you could not normally handle. Students earlier in their training do slow schedules down somewhat. The general positive effect the trainees will have for the individual physician as well as the general office staff will far outweigh the income issue.
   b. The status of a physician as a teacher will always result in a net gain of referrals.
5. It is important to provide opportunities for physicians to improve their skills as teachers, for we all feel more comfortable doing tasks at which we are more competent. Increasing comfort in ambulatory teaching will lessen resistance to students in the office.

Our teaching practice used the following program to help ourselves learn about teaching. Our group of eight doctors set up a monthly meeting to discuss and learn about teaching topics. At first, we met in the evening at 7:30 p.m. for 2 hours (at one of our homes). We now meet at 6 p.m. over a light dinner (in the office conference room). We choose the topic in advance, and one of us presents a topic of mutual concern, or we invite a knowledgeable guest to lead a discussion with us. Some of the topics have included the following:

- One-to-one teaching skills
- Small-group teaching skills
- Adult learning principles
- Direct observation techniques
- Learning theories
- Interaction with families

We also used our videotape facilities in these sessions. We bring tapes of various trainee encounters with patients and discuss ways of teaching the trainee in that situation. We may videotape ourselves teaching trainees, replay these tapes at the meetings, and provide comment and advice to each other on our teaching skills. These sessions have led us to understand the importance of improving our skills as teachers.

Additional Details

1. *Block versus longitudinal experiences:* There are two approaches to hav-ing trainees in your office: One is for an intensive experience during a short period (block time); the other is brief exposures during longer periods (longitudinal time). In block time, the trainee spends several weeks, or a month or two, working most of the day at the office. In longitudinal time, the trainee comes to the office for a specified period each week (i.e., one or two mornings or afternoons) during a period as long as a year. The rest of the time, the trainee rotates through other clinical disciplines or hospital wards.

    Which is ideal? Each has its advantages and disadvantages (Hershey, Reed, James, & Rosenthal, 1995). If block time is used, trainees are committed to a specific teaching site where they become familiar with the setting, its support staff, and patients. They quickly become fully integrated into the practice. There is a broad exposure to many prob-lems during a short period, and the students are available daily to the patients. There are few distractions to draw them away from the office. As the teachers get to know the trainees well and learn their strengths and weaknesses, the trainees may be given greater independence in their work and thus extend their learning experience (Steinweg, Cummings, & Kelly, 2001). The main disadvantage is that the trainee will be unable to observe the natural history of illness as well as learn about the appropriate follow-up of patients over the long term. Ambulatory block rotations have been successfully used in family medicine, primary care internal medicine, pediatrics, emergency medicine, and gynecology (Wisdom, Gruppen, Anderson, Grum, & Woolliscroft, 1993).

If longitudinal time is used, this kind of learning experience can be integrated with other rotations. Because trainees are involved with the clinic during a long period, they have the opportunity to follow patients regularly and learn about continuity of care, the natural history of illness, and appropriate follow-up intervals. More regular contact with the teacher seems to enhance learning and trainee satisfaction (Prislin et al., 1998). The major disadvantage is the scheduling problem: Conflicting service needs on inpatient units interfere with trainees getting away to the office. Longitudinal experiences have been used in many disciplines. They have been used successfully for medical student electives in early undergraduate years. Clerkships in primary care disciplines such as family medicine, pediatrics, and internal medicine have made wide use of this format. More recently, family medicine residency programs have made extensive use of the longitudinal model (Reust, 2001). Specialty disciplines such as obstetrics and gynecology, internal medicine, and surgical fields find this model attractive (Deutsch, 1997; Ogrine, Mutha, & Irby, 2002).

2. *Scheduling of patients with trainees:* There are several approaches to booking patients with trainees, depending on their stage of training and learning objectives.

   a. *Timing:* Early in their training, students take three to four times as long as an experienced clinician to see a patient. In addition, no two students or residents arrive with the same ability and level of experience. Thus, when trainees begin working at the office, allow them about an hour for a new patient and 30 minutes for follow-up visits. As you get a better idea of trainees' skills and as they improve with time, less time will be required. You may also want to build some extra time into your appointment bookings every fourth or fifth patient to allow for the inevitable discussion that will take place between patients (Whitehouse, Roland, & Campion, 1997).

   b. *Patient selection:* Early in their training trainees need to see more elementary clinical problems within the specialty. As they advance, give them more challenging cases. Exposure in early training to rare or complicated clinical presentations can lead to false impressions of disease prevalence and encourage exhaustive testing. Early exposure to patients with particularly difficult psychosocial issues can be overwhelming, leading trainees to feel less confident in their abilities to manage patient care (Smith & Irby, 1997).

In discussing their learning objectives, trainees will identify areas of weakness or special interest. Direct patients with these types of problems to them. Trainees should have their own section in the appointment book, and patients should be slotted in according to the learning needs and skill of the trainee. Otherwise, as patients come into the office, they can be selected out for the trainee to see, depending on their diagnosis.

c. *Specific booking:* In many ambulatory teaching settings, patients will be scheduled specifically to see trainees. This is important because trainees establish a roster of patients that recognize them as doctors and to whom they can provide continuous care. This may be less of an issue in specialty practices as opposed to primary care. Patients may not like it at first, but some teaching practices have been successful in offering earlier appointments to patients who are willing to deal with the trainee knowing that they will also get to see the teaching physician at that visit.

You will normally also be booked to see patients, and you will need time for teaching and perhaps some time to spend with the patient (Lesky & Hershman, 1995). There are many ways of accomplishing these tasks, taking into consideration the type of practice (specialty or primary care), personal preference, and the trainee's competence. One option is: Two patients are booked for the same time slot, with the next slot held open for supervision and teaching. In the third slot, a patient is booked for you, but the slot is held open for the student to do her own work. (This method preserves the total number of patients who would be seen without a student present and creates dedicated teaching time.) The student could complete the chart note and also spend time reading related material from textbooks in your office. Moreover, since many physicians have office-based computers with web access, trainees may use this time to search for relevant journal articles or clinical practice guidelines.

3. *Tracking:* It is helpful to both you and trainees to keep a log book of what types of patients trainees are seeing and perhaps what procedures they may have performed. This will assist trainees in evaluating their

learning plan and help you prepare for future students. With this information you can look for specific gaps in the trainees' experience and try to direct those types of patients to them. In addition, trainees may use this information when applying for hospital privileges upon graduation, if documentation of training experience is required. There are several methods that can be used:

a. In many practices, computerized billing systems are used. Use this to keep track of what your trainees see and do by making a notation in the computer of the trainee's name beside the billing doctor. With each billing entry, you have the sex, age, diagnosis, and any procedures for each patient. From these data, construct a profile of patients seen by each trainee according to diagnosis, age, sex, and the numbers of procedures performed by the trainee. Also, you can determine for the trainee whether patients return to see them on more than one occasion or choose to see someone else. You can also measure the trainee's ability to attract new patients. With a simple modification of the software, you can store number of patients seen, distribution of patients across diagnostic categories, and exposure to counseling or psychotherapy. Trainees may be compared against averages for all students coming to your practice. Trends may be observed from year to year. Any changes you make in the trainees' program may be monitored for their effect by reviewing practice profiles before and after the changes.

Here are some examples of profiles and their use. In Figure 3.6, a resident sees significantly fewer gynecology and obstetrical patients than the others in his group. In Figure 3.7, despite seeing fewer gynecology and obstetrical problems, this resident sees the same age-sex distribution of patients. Present these data to the resident and explore with him reasons for this discrepancy.

b. Trainees may complete their own record of learning by filling in a log sheet, which is often provided by the course director (Dolmans, Schmidt, van der Beek, Beintema, & Gerver, 1999). As they experience a clinical problem or procedure, they enter it onto the log record and keep a cumulative record. Figure 3.8 shows a sample of recording experience with common problems in primary care.

c. Computers can also be used for recording patient encounters and procedures performed. Using spreadsheet software on any desktop computer in your office, students can enter their patient encounters at a convenient point in the day. You could set up the spreadsheet to list the particular elements of your specialty. Hand-held personal

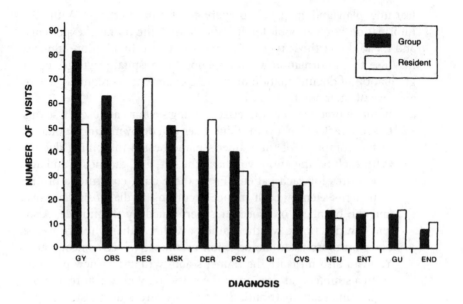

FIGURE 3.6   Diagnostic distribution, Resident J.

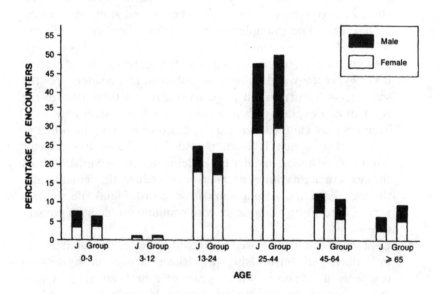

FIGURE 3.7   Age-sex distribution, Resident J.

Sample Patient Log Form

Common problems	Number Seen
Abdominal pain	① ② ③ ④ ⑤ ⑥
Alcohol abuse	① ② ③ ④ ⑤ ⑥
Arthritis	① ② ③ ④ ⑤ ⑥
Asthma	① ② ③ ④ ⑤ ⑥
Backache	① ② ③ ④ ⑤ ⑥
Cerebrovascular disease	① ② ③ ④ ⑤ ⑥
Contraception	① ② ③ ④ ⑤ ⑥
Chronic lung disease	① ② ③ ④ ⑤ ⑥
Depression/anxiety	① ② ③ ④ ⑤ ⑥
Diabetes mellitus	① ② ③ ④ ⑤ ⑥
Dizziness	① ② ③ ④ ⑤ ⑥
Drug abuse (legal/illegal)	① ② ③ ④ ⑤ ⑥
Earache	① ② ③ ④ ⑤ ⑥
Fatigue	① ② ③ ④ ⑤ ⑥
Headache	① ② ③ ④ ⑤ ⑥
Hypertension	① ② ③ ④ ⑤ ⑥
Insomnia	① ② ③ ④ ⑤ ⑥
Ischemic heart disease	① ② ③ ④ ⑤ ⑥
Skin rashes	① ② ③ ④ ⑤ ⑥
Sexually transmitted disease	① ② ③ ④ ⑤ ⑥
Upper respiratory infection	① ② ③ ④ ⑤ ⑥
Vaginitis	① ② ③ ④ ⑤ ⑥

Technical procedures	Number Performed
Immunizations	① ② ③ ④ ⑤ ⑥
Injections	① ② ③ ④ ⑤ ⑥
Syringing ears	① ② ③ ④ ⑤ ⑥
Cryotherapy of skin lesions	① ② ③ ④ ⑤ ⑥
Venipuncture	① ② ③ ④ ⑤ ⑥
Glucometer testing	① ② ③ ④ ⑤ ⑥

FIGURE 3.8   Sample patient log form.

digital assistants provide ready access for students to record encounters as the day proceeds (Bird, Zarum, & Renzi, 2001; Malan, Haffner, Armstrong, & Satin, 2000; Criswell & Parchman, 2002).

4. *Conflicting work loads:* Sometimes an ambulatory experience is viewed by the trainee as an add-on to an already busy rotation (e.g., a surgical intern spending two afternoons at a general surgeon's office in a longitudinal manner while assigned to a general surgery ward). The trainee finds that there is competition for his services. A trainee might be requested to scrub in at an emergency surgery or to complete a workup for an acutely ill patient in the emergency department. Ward rounds with the attending physician may interfere with time set aside for the office. At other times a trainee will be absent from the office because of a difficult night on call or the need to catch up on ward work or to prepare rounds. Some interruptions are unavoidable, but there are some strategies to minimize them.

   The program director must make it clear to all that the ambulatory care time has the same priority as everything else and must not get excluded because of other work routines.

   - The trainees' schedule, in cooperation with the dean's office, must be arranged to ensure adequate coverage for the hospital when trainees are scheduled for ambulatory care.
   - Trainees should adopt a buddy system whereby they team up in providing care and replace each other when in the office.
   - Physicians should work with trainees to help with time management so that trainees can learn the essential skills required for handling the tasks of a busy physician.

5. *Continuity of care:* In ambulatory care teaching, continuity of care in all specialties is an important learning objective. Continuity of care is defined as a series of interactions occurring over time by which the doctor is able to get a better picture of the patient over the course of her life or specific illness (Ruane & Brody, 1987). Continuity implies becoming an identified and trusted source of care for the patient. Learning issues for the trainee include (using hypertension as an example): the longevity of the diagnosis; previous attempted therapies and their success, failure, and side effects; definition of good control; frequency of follow-up visits; risk factors; and how often to order laboratory tests for target organ impact or medication side effects (Stearns & Glasser, 1993).

   Achieving this learning goal has several potential obstacles. These include the fact that the trainees are not on site every day, the rotation may be short, and the patient expects to be seen by the teaching physician (Roland, Mayor, & Morris, 1986). Students can be assisted with this learning goal by ensuring the following:

- Whenever possible, patients return to the same trainee for follow-up.
- Trainees have a defined roster of patients who remain their responsibility during the ambulatory experience.
- The office staff have the capacity to contact trainees when the trainees are away from the office. Then, the trainees will learn how to handle patient phone calls, new problems that have arisen or telling patients about abnormal laboratory results.
- The office staff contact the trainee for patient problems, understanding that this is an important educational activity for the student. Teaching physicians should resist dealing with a patient problem brought to them by the office staff and encourage them to take the extra time to contact the trainee while reemphasizing the importance of this extra step for the trainee's education.

6. *Patient consent for videotaping:* The extent of consent required from patients will vary according to the practice setting and individual circumstances. Most teaching practices outline the practice of direct observation in their patient information brochure as well as post a sign in each examination room (see page 41). In addition, written consent may be required, especially if any videotapes are kept past the time of the encounter. Figure 3.9 shows a sample consent form.

7. *Early undergraduate years:* Medical schools are moving some of the clinical teaching in the first few years of the curriculum from the bedside to the doctor's office. This includes the teaching of interviewing skills, history taking, physical examination, and clinical teaching within a specialty topic. Students are assigned to learn specific tasks: e.g., taking a medical history, practicing a lung examination, or learning cranial nerve testing. Even more creative planning is required to meet the learning needs of these students. (Much, of course, will depend on the number of students in each group.) Most medical schools still organize clinical teaching with chunks of prescheduled time (e.g., interviewing skills—Tuesday, 2–5 p.m.). You have little flexibility with the schedule, so you need to work with the time allotted. Try to do the following:

- Book patients from your volunteer register who have agreed to spend a few hours with students.

```
┌─────────────────────────────────────────────────────────────────┐
│                    VIDEOTAPE CONSENT FORM                         │
│                                                                   │
│ During your visit, a closed-circuit television system will be in  │
│ operation so that a teaching physician may watch from another     │
│ room.                                                             │
│                                                                   │
│ This is for the purpose of education to assist our trainees in    │
│ learning about interviewing patients.                             │
│                                                                   │
│ Strict confidentiality will be maintained.                        │
│                                                                   │
│ The conduct of the visit will be the same as usual, and the       │
│ viewing will not interfere in any way.                            │
│                                                                   │
│ If you prefer not to be involved, please inform your doctor, who  │
│ will switch off the system. Your decision not to participate      │
│ will in no way affect your care at the Clinics of Main Street.    │
│                                                                   │
│ I consent to the use of videotape recording during this visit     │
│ and for its review afterwards.                                    │
│ Date _____        Signature _____ │
└─────────────────────────────────────────────────────────────────┘
```

FIGURE 3.9   Sample videotape consent form.

- Schedule several follow-up visits of patients who might agree to spend time with a student as part of their appointment (Kurth, Irigoyen, & Schmidt, 1997).
- Arrange some new patients for that time slot who may agree to see one of the students voluntarily, especially if they are getting an earlier appointment than they would have with the usual waiting list.
- Have the student work with you during regular office time using a longitudinal model. Assign the student a specific task of history taking or physical examination so that only 15 to 20 minutes will be spent with the patient. Break the teaching into the very small chunks of time that are available between patients, instead of the usual lengthy time at the bedside with a captive patient.
- Stagger the time with patients to accommodate room availability and patient availability (especially when trying to get patients that demonstrate a particular clinical entity).

For example, during regular clinic time (2–5 p.m.), there are four students, two rooms, and two patients.

1:00 p.m.	Student A	Room 1	Patient X	Students C and D—
	Student B	Room 2	Patient Y	lunch
2:00 p.m.	Student C	Room 1	Patient X	Students A and B—
	Student D	Room 2	Patient Y	lunch
3:00 p.m.	Teaching time—office coffee room

- Arrange for one or two of the students to come to the office during other open time in their schedule when you have rooms or patients available. Then the students can use the scheduled clinic time for what had been planned for that open time (e.g., personal study, time off, etc.). Alternatively, use the scheduled clinical time for teaching with the entire assigned group of students, using patients previously seen in the office as the focus for discussion.

REFERENCES

Bird, S., Zarum, R., & Renzi, F. (2001). Emergency medicine resident patient care documentation using hand-held computerized device. *Academic Emergency Medicine, 8,* 1200–1203.

Carroll, J. C. (1986). The challenge of teaching obstetrics to family practice residents in a tertiary care hospital. *Canadian Family Physician, 32,* 2263–2265.

Criswell, D., & Parchman, M. (2002). Handheld computer use in U.S. family practice residency programs. *Journal of the American Medical Informatics Association, 9,* 80–86.

Deutsch, S. (1997). *Community-based teaching.* Philadelphia: American College of Physicians.

Dolmans, D., Schmidt, A., van der Beek, J., Beintema, M., & Gerver, W. (1999). Does a student log provide a means to better structure clinical education? *Medical Education, 33,* 89–94.

Grayson, M., Klein, M., Lugo, J., & Visintainer, P. (1998). Benefits and costs to community-based physicians teaching primary care to medical students. *Journal of General Internal Medicine, 13,* 485–488.

Hajioff, D., & Birchall, M. (1999). Medical students in ENT outpatient clinics: Appointment times, patient satisfaction and student satisfaction. *Medical Education, 33,* 669–673.

Hershey, C., Reed, P., James, P., & Rosenthal, T. (1995). Experience with community academic practice: Strategies for the ambulatory education of residents. *American Journal of Medicine, 99,* 536.

Kurth, R., Irigoyen, M., & Schmidt, H. (1997). A model to structure student learning in ambulatory care settings. *Academic Medicine, 72,* 601–606.

Lesky, L., & Hershman, W. (1995). Practical approaches to a major educational challenge: Training students in the ambulatory setting. *Archives of Internal Medicine, 155,* 897–904.

Malan, T., Haffner, W., Armstrong, A., & Satin, A. (2000). Hand-held computer operating system program for collection of resident experience data. *Obstetrics and Gynecology, 96,* 792–794.

Newton, J., Eccles, M., & Hutchinson, A. (1992). Communication between general practitioners and consultants: What should their letters contain? *British Medical Journal, 304,* 1181–1182.

Ogrine, G., Mutha, S., & Irby, D. (2002). Evidence for longitudinal ambulatory care rotations: A review of the literature. *Academic Medicine, 77,* 688–693.

Paulman, P., Susman, J., & Abboud, C. (2000). *Precepting medical students in the office.* Baltimore: Johns Hopkins University Press.

Prislin, M., Feighny, K., Stearns, J., Hood, J., Arnold, L., Erney, S., & Johnson, L. (1998). What students say about learning and teaching in longitudinal ambulatory primary care clerkships: A multi-institutional study. *Academic Medicine, 73,* 680–687.

Reust, C. (2001). Longitudinal residency training: A survey of family practice residency programs. *Family Medicine, 33,* 745.

Richards, R. (1996). *Building partnerships: Educating health professionals for the community they serve.* San Francisco: Jossey-Bass.

Roland, M., Mayor, V., & Morris, R. (1986). Factors associated with achieving continuity of care in general practice. *Journal of Royal College of General Practitioners, 36,* 102–104.

Ruane, T., & Brody, H. (1987). Understanding and teaching of continuity of care. *Journal of Medical Education, 62,* 96–97.

Simon, S., Peters, A., Christiansen, C., & Fletcher, R. (2000). Effect of medical student teaching on patient satisfaction in a managed care setting. *Journal of General Internal Medicine, 15,* 457–461.

Smith, S., & Irby, D. (1997). The roles of experience and reflection in ambulatory care education. *Academic Medicine, 72,* 32–35.

Stearns, J., & Glasser, M. (1993). How ambulatory care is different. *Medical Education, 27,* 35–40.

Steinweg, K., Cummings, D., & Kelly, S. (2001). Are some subjects better taught in block rotation? A geriatric experience. *Family Medicine, 33,* 756–761.

Tattersall, M., Griffin, A., Dunn, S., Monaghan, H., Scatchard, K., & Butow, P. (1995). Writing to referring doctors after a new patient consultation: What is wanted and what was contained in letters from one medical oncologist? *Australia and New Zealand Journal of Medicine, 25,* 463–464.

Whitehouse, C., Roland, M., & Campion, P. (1997). *Teaching medicine in the community.* Oxford: Oxford University Press.

Wisdom, K., Gruppen, L., Anderson, D., Grum, C., & Woolliscroft, J. (1993). Ambulatory-care-based education: Beyond the rhetoric. *Academic Medicine, 68,* s34–36.

—4—

Strategies to Use During the Teaching Day

During the weekly medical staff meeting at the Clinics of Main Street, Dr. Z. Z. Brown asked the director about the teaching function: "We now have all these students, interns, and residents working here almost every day. But there does not seem to be much teaching going on. Sure, we talk about the cases they see, but it's all rather spontaneous and haphazard. How can we make best use of our teaching time?"

Then Dr. Z. Z. Blue spoke: "Also, there are three obligations that have to be kept in mind in teaching practices: (a) the need for the attending physician to be responsible for care given by trainees and the obligation to review the trainee's work; (b) the need to maintain patient flow; and (c) the need to ensure patient satisfaction with high-quality care and continuity with their attending physician."

The director suggested that it is difficult to satisfy all of these concerns at the same time. It would be better to have some more time to discuss the various strategies the staff could use in their teaching day to help the trainees with their learning yet meet these requirements. They set a dinner meeting for the first Tuesday of the next month. The director suggested that they invite the associate dean of medical education, who was very knowledgeable about teaching strategies.

Here is a summary of the ideas that were generated.

TIMING

The day in the office is always busy for teachers who are seeing patients, answering telephone calls, dealing with consultants, referring doctors, or responding to office problems; there is never a dull moment. With lower reimbursement rates over the last decade, there has been an additional emphasis on clinical productivity in both academic centers and managed care practices (Ludmerer, 2000). When does the teaching fit in?

For every office and each doctor the answer will be different. It is important to plan your teaching activities so they are a scheduled part of the day rather than leaving them to chance. In a typical office day, the following are the most opportune moments:

1. In the morning, before the first patient—15 to 30 minutes for more concentrated teaching opportunities
2. Between each patient—a briefer time to review the salient points
3. At lunch—another chance to spend some relaxed time teaching
4. When a patient fails to show, and there is a gap in the day
5. After the last patient

TEACHING STRATEGIES

Table 4.1 lists various teaching strategies.

TABLE 4.1   Teaching Strategies Using Patients, Charts, and Educational Techniques

Patients	Charts	Educational Techniques
Case discussion	Chart review	Role play and simulation
Case review	Chart-stimulated recall	Short didactic presentation
Direct observation	Criterion chart review	

Use of Patients

During the day, as trainees see patients, you may use one of the following strategies:

•   Case discussion
•   Case review
•   Direct observation

Case Discussion: The following explains this strategy.

1. *Description:* This strategy is the most common one used in ambulatory care teaching. The trainee sees the patient first, and then presents the history, physical, and suggested management. The teacher usually asks the trainee some clarifying questions and then may see the patient to review the findings. Since the discussion occurs between patient visits and usually while the patient is still waiting, it will be brief and to the point. Thus you will make considerable use of responding and inquiry skills.

   To maintain patient flow, this will be a short encounter. For senior trainees, only a few minutes will usually suffice to clarify some teaching points. For junior trainees, 5 to 10 minutes may be required to review the case, see the patient, and highlight some management issues before the patient leaves.

2. *Indications:* This strategy is best used with the inexperienced learner when direct observation is unavailable. It is also important to use when patients also see the attending physician. It allows for closer control with newer trainees and also diminishes students' anxiety, for they know that you will be available for consultation.

3. *Advantages:* The following are advantages of this strategy.

   - Close monitoring of the trainee
   - Fulfillment of the legal obligation to review the patient
   - Evaluation of trainee's knowledge and decision making by listening to case presentation
   - Quick suggestions on patient management

4. *Limitations:* The following are limitations of this strategy.

   - Reliance mainly on the students' report of the case
   - Limited to assessment of cognitive domain
   - Restriction of autonomy of the learner who has more experience
   - Technique more time consuming than case review because each case is discussed between patients

5. *Cost:* The following items refer to time and resources.

   - Economical strategy (i.e., one teacher can supervise two or three students)
   - Requires no equipment
   - Teacher may see patients simultaneously

6. *Example:* You are the emergency physician on duty. An intern has just finished taking a history on a patient with acute abdominal pain. From listening to his case presentation, you surmise that he has focused on a diagnosis of renal colic and ignored the points in the history about possible gastrointestinal pathology. At this point you tell him about this deficiency in history taking and ask him to report the rest after he has completed his physical examination.

7. *Tips:* The following tips are helpful when using this strategy.
   a. Keep track of points that may come up in the brief discussion between patients for fuller discussion at lunch or later in the day. Carry a small pad in your pocket to make these notes.
   b. Remember the teachable moment.
   c. Resist the urge to cover everything. Be brief, and do not contribute to the trainee falling further behind. This is not the one and only time the trainee will see a specific case—make one or two points (Smith & Irby, 1997; Baldwin, 1997) and leave the rest to another opportunity that you or another teacher will surely find.

Case Review: The following explains this strategy.

1. *Description:* This method of reviewing a larger number of cases at one sitting can be used at lunchtime or the end of the day. Sitting down with one or more trainees who are working in the office, the teacher asks each one to present the history and physical examination to the group. The teacher then leads a discussion based on the case presented. Many cases can be reviewed without lengthy discussion. Others merit more careful scrutiny and analysis. Finally, you may choose one topic generated by one of the cases for more lengthy discussion. These sessions may last from $1/2$ to 1 hour, depending on time availability (Mcdonagh, 1997).

2. *Indications:* This method is best used when you are in a clinical environment with experienced trainees who benefit from more autonomy (i.e., not having to review each case directly after the patient is seen). It is also preferred when patient flow does not allow time to discuss each case at the time of the visit.

3. *Advantages:* The following are advantages of this strategy.

   • Fulfills legal obligations of patient review by licensed physician
   • Increases learner autonomy by maintaining supervision at a distance
   • Allows more in-depth evaluation of student's knowledge base

4. *Limitations:* The following are limitations of this strategy.

   - Does not assess physical examination or interviewing skills
   - Depends on student's account of the encounter
   - Causes more anxiety for beginning learner

5. *Cost:* The following points are related to the cost of this method.

   - Protects income for the practice because teacher can continue to see patients (albeit at a reduced number) while trainees work simultaneously
   - Extra time needs to be set aside for a teaching session after patients are seen

6. *Example:* Over lunch, you and two residents working in the office sit down in your office to review all patients seen that morning. Each case is presented one by one with only a brief review. One resident presents a problem patient with chronic obstructive pulmonary disease. You then all agree to discuss at length the topic of steroid use in chronic lung disease. This discussion lasts for about 15 minutes, after which you review the remainder of their cases briefly.

7. *Tips:* The following tips are helpful when using this strategy.
   a. Remember the principles of adult learning and the trainees' personal learning plan. At the outset ask the students if they have some topic they wish to cover, especially one raised by a case seen that day. Use the other trainees present, particularly seniors, to contribute to the teaching.
   b. Remember to tell the learners how well they are functioning (e.g., "that was well managed because . . . " or "your understanding of the physiology is excellent"). You are making judgments all the time as the students present cases and discuss topics. Let them know how they are doing (Schwenk & Whitman, 1993).
   c. Present some of the cases you've seen to add important clinical material and to enhance the collegial atmosphere.
   d. If it was a rather mundane day and you draw a blank on a good topic for discussion, use the "wheel of fortune." Take one case of the day, put the diagnosis or presenting complaint at the hub of a wheel drawing, and ask those present to give a related topic to complete each spoke (see Figure 4.1). There are now several topics from which to choose.
   e. At this session your skill of asking questions will be used most. Use questions to stimulate discussion rather than to provide infor-

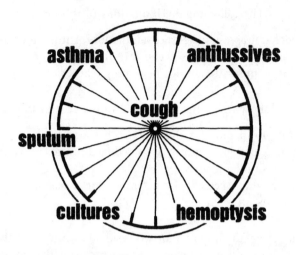

FIGURE 4.1   Sample "wheel" with presenting complaint at center and related topics completing each spoke.

mation. Use questions that require interpretation rather than factual answers (Jacques, 1992). Rather than say "Describe the use of steroids in COPD," try "How does the idea that steroids reduce inflammation apply to the treatment of COPD?"

f.   Be patient when there is no response to your question. Get used to silence. It gives time for the student to reflect on the question, or for peers to help. It also discourages overcompetitiveness to see who can shout out the answer first (Tiberius, 1995).

g.   Involve all the trainees in the group by directing questions to the rest of the group or to each individual: "What do the rest of you think?" "Isn't that similar to what you were saying earlier, Joanne?" (Westberg & Jason, 1996; Mackway-Jones & Walker, 1999).

h.   Begin the discussion with a controversial statement to cause disagreement. A certain degree of surprise or uncertainty arouses curiosity, a basic motive to learn (McKeachie, 1986). For example: "From your case of Mrs. M, the 50-year-old patient here today for the periodic health exam, I believe that all postmenopausal women at risk for osteoporosis should be on hormonal replacement therapy indefinitely—Agree?"

Direct Observation: The following explains this strategy.

1. *Description:* Direct observation can be accomplished by using a video camera, seeing through a one-way glass, or sitting in the consultation room with the learner. The teacher can actively participate in the encounter by making suggestions to the learner via a telephone intercom. The learner can also check with the teaching physician by stepping out of the room at a prearranged time (e.g., before doing the physical examination, while the patient is undressing).

   Videotape is now the preferred technology of direct observation. The tape can be reviewed later when more time is available. While watching the tape, the learner can observe his or her interviewing skills (both verbal and nonverbal) and review attitudes and feelings about the patient. These and other issues observed by the teacher can then be discussed (Premi, 1991).

   We have used the following equipment in our office.

   - Black-and-white surveillance camera, with wide-angle lens, mounted on a supporting bracket (used by stores for theft prevention)
   - VHS videocassette recorder
   - Twenty-inch television set
   - Pressure zone microphone (we place ours directly in the ceiling, not hanging down from it, by cutting a small hole in the soft tiles); most suppliers will install the equipment at a cost of about $1,000.

2. *Indications:* This strategy is best used for supervision and teaching of interviewing skills, physical examination, organizational skills, clinical reasoning, and attitudes (Westberg & Jason, 1994).

3. *Advantages:* The following are advantages of this strategy.

   - Fulfills legal obligation for patient supervision as well as for teaching about clinical knowledge, decision making, and interviewing
   - Obviates the need for learner to repeat the details of the history and physical before you discuss management
   - Provides opportunity, with videotape, for learners to see what they have done and draw some of their own conclusions; teacher's points can be seen instead of just described (Campbell, Howie, & Murray, 1995)

4. *Limitations:* The following are limitations of this method.

   - Time-consuming
   - Increase in learners' anxiety, knowing they are being watched
   - Presence of teacher in room often interferes with relationship between student and patient
   - Use of videotape requires patient consent

5. *Cost:* The following are related to the cost of this strategy.

   - Moderate expense for equipment
   - Process of sitting in with learner reduces number of patients you see
   - If session is videotaped, you can continue to see patients during office hours, but time is set aside later for review of tape (this time may be at the expense of other practice activities)

6. *Example:* A second-year medical student is in your office for her clinical experience in cardiology. You have arranged to see two patients from your volunteer register. As you see some of your follow-up patients, the student interviews these two patients and videotapes the encounters. Afterward, you watch both histories with her. She has been having trouble in previous visits to your office in completing the history in a reasonable time. On the tapes, you can both see that she is uncertain of the sequence of questions, gets quite confused, and goes in circles around the presenting complaint. You then discuss how she might learn to question the patient in a more efficient manner.

7. *Tips:* The following tips are helpful when using this strategy.

   a. You may not know what to look for when you start using direct observation (Cox & Mulholland, 1993). Figure 4.2 shows a cue sheet that may be used to help guide your observation as well as provide a space where you can make notes to remember significant points for comment. This way you can provide specific examples of your points instead of generalities, especially when you do not have videotape equipment.

   b. If using a videotape machine, watch the counter, and note when interesting interactions happen with the patient so you do not have to replay the entire tape. Choose one or two of these segments to review when only a brief time is available.

   c. Remember your skill in using a learner premise. You will use this skill in direct observation.

DIRECT OBSERVATION ENCOUNTER FORM		

NAME _____   DATE _____

Rating   4 - above current level of training   3 - satisfactory for level of training
         2 - below level of training   1 - unsatisfactory

	Score	Examples
INTERVIEWING SKILLS		
• *Introduction* (introduces self, puts patient at ease)		
• *Techniques* (mixes open and closed questions, listens to patient)		
• *Vocabulary* (avoids medical jargon, clear explanations)		
• *Closure* (explains diagnosis clearly, allows patient questions)		
HISTORY		
• *Problem definition* (identifies main reason for visit, full details of problem, picks up non-verbal cues)		
• *Comprehensiveness* (complete history when appropriate, avoids unnecessary detail)		
DOCTOR-PATIENT RELATIONSHIP		
• *Response to patient* (empathy, support)		
• *Respect for patient* (acts in professional manner, drapes patient properly)		

Suggestions _____
_____
_____
_____

FIGURE 4.2   Direct Observation Encounter Form.

    d. Let the tape roll, and ask the learner to stop it when he or she feels like making a comment or asking a question about an issue of concern. Otherwise, stop the tape occasionally and ask the learner for comments first before you give your opinion.

Use of Charts

The completion of the chart or electronic medical record of the visit is an essential part of each patient encounter. It can also be valuable when teaching in the ambulatory care setting. There are three ways that the chart can become an integral part of your office teaching:

- Chart review
- Chart-stimulated recall
- Criterion chart review

Chart Review: The following explains this strategy.

1. *Description:* This strategy is very similar to case review, but the written or electronic record of the patient's visit is used instead of the learner's verbal report (Morrell, 1981). At lunchtime, the end of the day, or any other convenient block of approximately 30 minutes, you can sit down to review the previous session's patients. Chart by chart, you read the trainee's entry of the visit, the history and physical, the diagnosis, the tests ordered, and treatment recommendations. You may follow this with discussion on the essentials of completing charts as well as on any other topic generated by the case at issue, either from the teacher- or learner-based premise. You could also cover basic items like legibility, format, length, thoroughness, problem-based summary sheets, electronic templates, and preparation of consultation reporting letters.
2. *Indications:* This strategy is best used with more senior trainees who will have worked more or less autonomously during the patient session, but there is a requirement for patient review at the end of the session. Alternatively, with students or junior trainees (where you have already reviewed each case before the patient left), this strategy can be used to focus on the teaching of the written record.
3. *Advantages:* The following are advantages of this strategy.

   - Fulfills legal obligations for review of case by licensed physician
   - Ensures quality of written record

- Is less dependent on trainee's verbal report
- Uses case material for discussion and teaching
- Allows for teaching of chart writeup or use of electronic medical record systems

4. *Limitations:* The following are disadvantages of this strategy.

   - Depends on trainee's written report of encounter
   - Does not assess interviewing or physical examination skills

5. *Cost:* The following are related to the cost of this strategy.

   - Interferes little with practice routine
   - Time is set aside for teaching after patients are seen

6. *Example:* A resident is working in the outpatient clinic this month. He has seen his list of patients for the morning, and you sit down to review his cases. One by one, you read each chart and discuss the case management with him as well as some topics of concern to him that are inspired by several of the cases. After completing the charts, it is apparent to you that he did not have a clear, organized format for completing the charts, even though he seems to get all the important information on the record. You then spend the last 10 minutes of the 30-minute session developing with him a system with which he feels comfortable, based on the SOAP (Subjective Objective Assessment Plan) format.

7. *Tips:* The following tips are helpful when using this strategy.
   a. Remember the teachable moment. The patient's record visually highlights issues on which a lasting impression can be made.
   b. The fact that you use the chart as a teaching stimulator will give the learner a strong message about the importance of the patient's record.
   c. Reviewing charts is an important tool in developing quality assurance programs for ambulatory care settings. If you make chart review part of your teaching, trainees will gain insight into how health care can be improved through chart audit.

Chart-Stimulated Recall: The following explains this strategy.

1. *Description:* Use this strategy in a one-to-one session with a learner working in your office. Choose a time when you have at least 30 minutes. Ask the learner to select several charts of patients she has

seen. Randomly select two charts to cover in the next 30 minutes. Give the learner one of the charts and ask her to review and recall the patient encounter in a stepwise fashion (Norman et al., 1989).

Use the chart to spur the memory of the learner to recall not only what happened with that particular case but also her thinking during the encounter. Asks questions, like the following:

"What were you thinking at that point?"
"Why did you ask those questions?"
"What led you to that conclusion?"
"Why did you stop there?"
"What other things were you thinking of?"
"Did you have a most likely diagnosis at that point?"
"Why choose those options?"

Do this for each stage of the interview (i.e., history, physical examination, differential diagnosis, severity of illness, etiology, plan of action, and choice of investigation and treatment). Enquire at each of these steps as to what the learner was thinking before she moved on to the next. Encourage the learner to explore her thinking process during the interview and not in retrospect after its completion (Reinhart & Keef, 1990; Solomon, Reinhart, Bridgham, Munger, & Starnaman, 1990).

2. *Indications:* This strategy is used to evaluate and assist learners in understanding and improving their clinical reasoning or decision-making process (Barrows, 1985). It is especially helpful for learners who seem disorganized in the patient encounters, have poor time management, are constantly behind, or cannot seem to make a firm decision.

3. *Advantages:* The following are advantages of this strategy.

    *   Powerful strategy for reviewing decision-making processes because time is set aside for this purpose, and the focus is entirely on the thought processes rather than getting caught up in management issues
    *   Chart provides stimulus to recall details of what actually occurred

4. *Limitations:* The following are limitations of this strategy.

    *   Is time consuming
    *   Requires that specific time be set aside in addition to time used for routine review of the patients seen
    *   Has to be done within a limited time after the patients have been seen, probably within 48 hours
    *   Is initially anxiety provoking for the learner and requires a lot of trust between learner and teacher

5. *Cost:* The following are related to the cost of this strategy.

    - Extra time needs to be set aside in addition to regular patient supervision.
    - This time is at expense of regular practice activities or other personal time

6. *Example:* A final-year medical student is doing a required rotation in your office. You see each patient with him after he has seen the patient. He seems to take forever with each patient. Although he gets a good grasp of his patient's problems, he is very slow. You decide to sit down with him after you have finished seeing all the patients for the day. You ask him to select four interesting charts from the previous 2 days and bring them to your office. At the session you go through the chart-stimulated recall procedure with two of those charts. It becomes apparent that each time John sees a patient he keeps asking more and more questions to confirm the hypothesis that he is formulating in his mind (i.e., he keeps seeking more clues in the decision tree). No wonder he takes so long with each patient. The two of you plan to review the cases again to see where he could have shortened the searching for cues yet still felt comfortable that his hypothesis was confirmed. You also decide that next week, when he is presenting his cases to you, he will alert you to when in the interview his main hypothesis first came to mind to help him further improve on shortening the search for confirmation.

7. *Tips:* The following tips are helpful when using this strategy.
    a. This type of strategy is used only on an occasional basis and usually not more than once every 2 weeks.
    b. It is used not only for learners with problems but may also be used with high-functioning learners to teach them the process of decision making.
    c. The procedure can also be used with videotapes of the learner's encounters. Run the tape, asking the learner to interrupt at any point to tell you what he was thinking. Question the learner about his thoughts as you see fit. The videotape replay acts as a potent stimulus to recall what was going on in the learner's thinking.

Criterion Chart Review: The following explain this strategy.

1. *Description:* This is another strategy for completing a chart review (Tugwell & Dok, 1985). It differs in that you audit the charts on your own, at your own pace, when you can set aside about 15 to 30 minutes. Provide the results to the learner at a session the following day. A

standard checklist acts as a guide to what to look for in the chart. It is an efficient and reliable method for reviewing the student's ability in taking a complete and comprehensive medical history (Woolliscroft, Calhoun, Beauchamp, Wolf, & Maxim, 1984).

A good project for you and your colleagues is to draw up a checklist of your own (Paccione, Cohen, & Schwartz, 1989). You can use one of your evening sessions to discuss what information you think is most important to gather from the chart and draw up a one-page sheet to use during the chart review. It can be typed and photocopied for use by your group members. Going through the process of creating the checklist will assist all of you to better understand the strategy of criterion chart review.

The checklist varies somewhat according to specialty, but there are basic elements to every patient encounter. Figure 4.3 gives an example from our practice.

2. *Indications:* Use this strategy to review patients seen by the trainees working in your office when there is little time to meet with trainees during the usual work day. Review the trainee's work in your spare time and away from the trainee.

3. *Advantages:* The following are advantages of this strategy.

- Fulfills medical legal requirement for review of patient by licensed physician
- Ensures quality of patient's record
- Can be deferred to chosen time
- Checklist provides stimulus for teacher to recall specific criticisms
- Provides descriptive information to the learner on the patient management and chart writeup
- Permits senior trainee to work autonomously and be evaluated subsequently
- Takes less time than direct observation, but you can gather a fair amount of information for teaching (Woolliscroft et al., 1984)

4. *Limitations:* The following are limitations of this strategy.

- Requires more time than other chart review methods because of your independent scrutiny of the charts followed by a meeting with the learner to give her a summary of your review
- Depends largely on trainee's record of encounter
- Does not assess interviewing or physical examination skills

CRITERION CHART REVIEW FORM

NAME _____ DATE _____

Rating 3 - exceeds expectations   2 - meets expectations
        1 - below expectations   0 - missing from chart

Criterion	Score	Comments
PRESENTING PROBLEM		
• main reason for visit clearly identified		
• full description of problem with relevant detail including pertinent negative questions		
HEALTH REVIEW		
• lists ongoing medical problems, previous surgery, medications, allergies, immunizations & major health risks		
FAMILY HISTORY		
• details of 1st degree relatives written on genogram		
PROBLEM FORMULATION		
• main problem accurately identified		
• comprehensive list of patient's problems		
MANAGEMENT PLAN		
• investigations appropriate to costs, risks and prevalence; correct treatment prescribed; if referral, appropriate?		
LEGIBILITY		
• able to read handwriting without difficulty		
OVERALL ORGANIZATION		
• uses S.O.A.P. format, patient profile sheet completed		

FIGURE 4.3   Criterion Chart Review Form.

5. *Cost:* The following is related to the cost of this strategy.

    • Requires considerable time for preparation of checklist and the
      actual chart review, but not at the expense of practice income

6. *Example:* A senior resident is assigned to your specialty group and
   works independently. At night, you review the charts prepared by her.
   Using your checklist, you note that she is documenting everything
   appropriately and has managed all her cases well but enters scant
   details of the history and physical. You note some examples on the
   checklist and meet with her just before you do hospital rounds the
   next day to review the checklist.

7. *Tip:* The following tips are helpful when using this strategy.
    a. Give the blank checklist to the trainee when she first starts at your
        office so that she is aware of what you are looking for when doing
        a criterion chart review. Then it is not a surprise examination, but
        a planned learning experience.
    b. In the ambulatory setting, rounds similar to inpatient attending
        rounds are difficult to establish. If there are more than one trainee
        assigned to your clinic, meet with them in the morning for an
        ambulatory morning report. Use cases drawn from the criterion
        chart review as a basis for a comprehensive review of one or two
        topics (Malone & Jackson, 1993). Invite other staff doctors from
        your clinic to present a case of interest (Wright & Helliwell, 1991).

Use of Educational Techniques

Sometimes, patients do not provide the necessary case material for teaching.
Here are several strategies that may be used when time is short, that require
limited preparation, and that can be used to focus learning on a particular
topic. They are the following:

• Role play and simulation
• Short didactic presentation

Role Play and Simulation: The following explains these strategies.

1. *Description:* Role play is the acting out of a defined character in a mock
   situation. Individuals take the parts of the doctor and patient, and
   attempt to recreate an office visit. Usually, the teacher plays the role
   of a patient and acts out a particular scene or medical problem while
   the learner conducts an interview. It is also useful, however, to have

the student play the patient or have students play both roles, if more than one learner is present (Siegel, 1998).

Use actual patient encounters as the material for the role play. When the student plays the doctor, have her practice different parts of the interview and various approaches to each circumstance. Follow each segment with a sharing of comments from both players about the effectiveness of the approach and their underlying feelings about the role (Mackway-Jones & Walker, 1999).

Role play can be open or structured.

Open: The patient role is played following intuition and previous experience with patients.
Structured: The player follows a specific script so that a very definite learning point can be made (Littlefield, Hahn, & Meyer, 1999).

Some medical schools have actors or other interested people rehearse to play clinical scenarios. These people are specially trained to simulate a patient in every detail. They can reproduce a patient's problem as if it were their own and present the same physical and emotional picture as the actual patient (Barrows & Tamblyn, 1980).

Simulated patients provide for the teacher a consistent, identified patient problem that can be scheduled for a convenient time. These simulated patients can provide unbiased feedback to students about their own reactions to the interview (Norman, Barrows, Gliva, & Woodward, 1985).

Banks of simulated patients are usually developed through the dean's office of the medical school. They are often included in part of the curriculum for teaching interviewing skills and could be used effectively in an actual office setting to add some reality to the simulation.

Role-play teaching can be set aside for a prearranged time (20–25 minutes are required). It can also be used spontaneously in the course of an informal case discussion, when a learning point could best be understood with this type of simulation. If you have the facility, record the simulation (Steinert, 1993).

2. *Indications:* Use this strategy to help trainees to recognize and focus on difficulties in interviewing, history taking, psychotherapy, patient education, or dealing with difficult patients such as those who are angry, flirtatious, or withdrawn. The technique can also be used as preparation for board or licensing examinations.

3. *Advantages:* The following are advantages of this strategy.

   - Interviewing is done under controlled, safe circumstances. The unplanned and uncontrolled variability of patients can be eliminated.

- The learner can receive an immediate response and actually try corrective strategies without fear of upsetting patients.
- There is not the time pressure of an office schedule.
- By playing the patient, the student can experience what it is like to be in the patient's place and gain valuable insight into her own attitudes.

4. *Limitations:* The following are limitations of this strategy.

- Trainees often complain that the simulation is not real and that the artificiality interferes with their usual performance. This response reflects the anxiety of the trainee. It is our experience that the performance in simulations is remarkably consistent with that of "real" patients.
- It can be very anxiety provoking for the trainee to try to play the role of a particular patient.
- For the strategy to succeed, the teacher and learner must trust each other.

5. *Cost:* The following are related to the cost of this strategy.

- Time needs to be set aside in addition to regular patient supervision.
- If using simulated patients, you need to coordinate with your medical school to bring the actors to the office.

6. *Example:* You are working with a junior resident in your office this month. Some patients have complained about his bedside manner. You note, however, that the difficulties arise mainly with your most demanding patients. You set up a time at lunch the next day to do a role-play session with the resident in which you play a demanding patient. During the role play, it is obvious that the resident reacts angrily at the first indication that this patient may be overly demanding. You discuss with him this reaction and the reasons behind it, as well as possible options in dealing with this kind of patient.

Short Didactic Presentation: The following explains this strategy.

1. *Description:* This is a traditional method of teaching in medicine. One person presents information to others, typically covering a cognitive area of learning. Either teacher or trainee may present a brief topic pertaining to the ambulatory care rotation, usually in response to

an interesting or difficult patient. We have found that a 10-minute presentation is sufficient to provide a concise summary of the material and prevent overloading the students with unnecessary detail. In our office, these presentations are usually done as part of a case review session at lunchtime or at the end of the workday.

2. *Indications:* This strategy is used when there is a well-defined gap in knowledge in a given clinical area. It may also be used to cover any core topics required by the curriculum in your medical school. As trainees in ambulatory experiences encounter a variable and random mix of patients, supplemental structured time may be required to enhance their breadth of knowledge of common ambulatory problems. This strategy could also be used for teaching about practice management, writing consultation reports to referring physicians, time management in the office, or billing matters.

3. *Advantages:* The following are advantages of this strategy.

   - Provokes less anxiety than other methods, for there is time to prepare in advance
   - Covers topic concisely
   - Gives trainees opportunity to practice presentation skills and get comments from you
   - Shows trainees how members of a group in practice can help each other keep up to date on knowledge and skills

4. *Limitations:* The following are limitations of this strategy.

   - Is useful mainly for cognitive areas of learning
   - Requires advanced preparation in spare time

5. *Cost:* The following is related to the cost of this strategy.

   - Brief addition of time to your regular teaching and supervision of patient care

6. *Example:* The course director for your specialty asks that you cover six specific common problems with trainees at your clinic. You ask your two trainees to prepare three topics each to be presented at a case review session held twice weekly.

7. *Tips:* The following tips are helpful when using this strategy.

   a. Use the patients discussed at case review sessions to generate topics for short didactic presentations. Assign a topic or specific reading to a trainee and set a mutually agreeable time for its presentation.

If the presentation is not part of regularly scheduled rounds, mark it on your calendar; otherwise, you will forget about it.

b. When conducting a short didactic presentation, do the following:

- Break the information down into easily assimilated components.
- Try to relate the information to previously learned material.
- Aim for the trainees current level of knowledge and build on that.
- Keep the amount of information limited to between three to six units of knowledge.

c. To use a problem-based learning method, provide the trainees with an actual patient example of a core topic and ask them to build their presentation from that case (Lawrence, Grosenick, Simpson, & Van Susteren, 1992; David, Patel, Burdett, & Rangachari, 1999).

d. Guide your trainees to prepare these presentations as a model of continued learning within the time constraints of real world practice. Evidence-based clinicians of the future do not need to be experts in clinical epidemiology, but they need to know how to manage high-quality knowledge products (Guyatt, Meade, Jaeschke, Cook, & Haynes, 2000). There are now many excellent distillation services that present the busy practitioner with preappraised evidence resources (Evans, 2001). Clinical practice guidelines are widely available for topics in many specialties. This information can all be accessed via paper journals or web-based sources using desktop computers or hand-held devices (Shaughnessy, Slawson, & Becker, 1998; Criswell & Parchman, 2002). Demonstrate to your trainee how you access these resources, depending on your own personal comfort level with the various technologies (Speedie, Pacala, & Vercellotti, 2001).

e. It is difficult to ensure that core topics of the curriculum are covered during the ambulatory experience. One of the trainees may be on vacation, have conflicting inpatient responsibilities, or have post night-call duties and thus may be away from your office just when you have scheduled a core topic discussion. To avoid unnecessary repetition, store the content of the presentation (either in a word-processing document or in Powerpoint slides) on a disk or your office computer. The trainees can then access and review the content at their convenience. You can even use e-mail or web-based storage sites (either the medical school's website or

inexpensive private storage sites) so that trainees may access the
seminar material and related background reading from a remote
site.

A COMMENT ON COST

At the conclusion of the dinner meeting to discuss all these teaching
strategies, Dr. Brown again had a question: "Sure, we can use all these
good educational strategies, but what will it cost us? What are the financial
implications for our practice to be an ambulatory care teaching center?"

Based on the current literature, Dr. Smith can comfortably report the
following to his colleagues:

- There is no difference in billed charges when trainees are present
  (Fields, Toffler, & Bledsoe, 1994). Some practices that were long-
  standing training sites actually reported an increase in billings when
  students were present (Adams & Eisenberg, 1997).
- There may be a slight decrease in productivity, that is, in the number
  of patients seen by the teaching physician (Kearl & Mainous, 1993).
  This seems to average about two patients per day, with some slightly
  larger numbers reported by offices where managed care has a
  larger role.
- Physicians do spend a longer time in the office when trainees are
  present (average of about 30 minutes daily) (Vinson, Paden, Devera-
  Sales, Marshall, & Waters, 1997; Doyle & Patricoski, 1997; Levy,
  Gjerde, & Albrecht, 1997), but they do this because it increases
  their enjoyment of the practice of medicine and leads to activities
  that further professional growth, such as increased reading of the
  medical literature and reviewing the basics of clinical medicine
  (Grayson, Klein, Lugo, & Visintainer, 1998; Dodson, 1998; Boex et
  al., 2000).

Figure 4.4 presents a summary chart that lists all the strategies, as well
as their indications, advantages, limitations, and relative cost, in a form
for easy comparison.

TEACHING STRATEGIES - SUMMARY

STRATEGY	INDICATIONS	ADVANTAGES	LIMITATIONS	COST
case discussion	- new trainee - quick suggestions between patients	• close monitoring of trainee	• relies on trainee report	• economical • teacher works simultaneously
case review	- experienced trainee	• increased trainee autonomy	• relies on trainee report	• income protected as teacher and trainee work simultaneously
	- patient flow does not allow for discussion between cases	• in-depth evaluation of knowledge		• extra time required for teaching after patients seen
direct observation	- teaching interviewing skills, physical exam, clinical reasoning & attitudes	• no need to report details of history • learner draws own conclusions from viewing tape	• learner anxiety • specific patient consent required • time consuming	• expensive for equipment & review time
chart review	- senior trainees	• not dependent on verbal report	• relies on written record	• inexpensive as patient time not interrupted
	- teaching about written record		• learning only in cognitive domain	• time spent after patients to review charts
chart stimulated recall	- teaching about decision making	• chart is stimulus to recall events	• time consuming	• sacrifice of after patient hours
criterion chart review	- detailed review of learner's knowledge	• deferred to convenient time	• time consuming • relies on written record	• time consuming but not at the expense of practice income
role play	- focussed teaching of interviewing skills, attitudes	• controlled circumstances	• anxiety provoking • ?artificial	• time required in addition to regular patient review
short didactic presentation	- learning in cognitive domain	• covers topic efficiently • low anxiety level	• advanced preparation	• efficient use of time during the day

FIGURE 4.4   Summary of teaching strategies.

REFERENCES

Adams, M., & Eisenberg, J. (1997). What is the cost of ambulatory education? *Journal of General Internal Medicine, 12,* S104–110.

Baldwin, L. (1997). Managing clinic time while precepting medical students. *Family Medicine, 29,* 13.

Barrows, H. (1985). *How to design a problem-based curriculum for the pre-clinical years.* New York: Springer Publishing.

Barrows, H., & Tamblyn, R. (1980). *Problem-based learning: An approach to medical education.* New York: Springer Publishing.

Boex, J., Boll, A., Franzini, L., Hogan, A., Irby, D., Merservey, P., Rubin, R., Seifer, S., & Veloski, J. (2000). Measuring the costs of primary care education in the ambulatory setting. *Academic Medicine, 75,* 419–425.

Campbell, L., Howie, J., & Murray, S. (1995). Use of videotaped consultations in summative assessment of trainees in general practice. *British Journal of General Practice, 45,* 137–141.

Cox, J., & Mulholland, H. (1993). An instrument for assessment of videotapes of general practitioners' performance. *British Medical Journal, 306,* 1043–1046.

Criswell, D., & Parchman, M. (2002). Handheld computer use in U.S. family practice residency programs. *Journal of the American Medical Informatics Association, 9,* 80–85.

David, T., Patel, L., Burdett, K., & Rangachari, P. (1999). *Problem-based learning in medicine.* Lake Forest, IL: Royal Society of Medicine Press.

Dodson, M. (1998). Motivation and reward factors that affect private physician involvement in an obstetrics and gynecology clerkship. *Obstetrics and Gynecology, 4,* 628–632.

Doyle, G., & Patricoski, C. (1997). Costs of teaching for community teachers in family medicine. *Family Medicine, 29,* 12–13.

Evans, M. (2001). Creating knowledge management skills in primary-care residents. *American College of Physicians Journal Club,* September/October, 2001, A-11-12.

Fields, S., Toffler, W., & Bledsoe, N. (1994). Impact of the presence of a third-year medical student in gross charges and patient volumes in 22 rural community practices. *Academic Medicine, 69,* S87–89.

Grayson, M., Klein, M., Lugo, J., & Visintainer, P. (1998). Benefits and costs to community-based physicians teaching primary care to medical students. *Journal of General Internal Medicine, 13,* 485–488.

Guyatt, G., Meade, M., Jaeschke, R., Cook, D., & Haynes, R. (2000). Practitioners of evidence based care. Not all clinicians need to appraise evidence from scratch but all need some skills. *British Medical Journal, 320,* 954–955.

Jacques, D. (1992). *Learning in groups* (2nd ed.). Houston: Gulf Publishing Company.

Kearl, G., & Mainous, A. (1993). Physicians' productivity and teaching responsibilities. *Academic Medicine, 2,* 166–167.

Lawrence, S., Grosenick, D., Simpson, D., & Van Susteren, T. (1992). A comparison of problem-based and didactic approaches to learning on an ambulatory medicine clerkship. *Teaching and Learning in Medicine, 4,* 221–224.

Levy, B., Gjerde, C., & Albrecht, L. (1997). The effects of precepting on and the support desired by community-based preceptors in Iowa. *Academic Medicine, 72,* 382–384.

Littlefield, J., Hahn, H., & Meyer, A. (1999). Evaluation of a role-play learning exercise in an ambulatory setting. *Advances in Health Sciences Education, 4,* 167–173.

Ludmerer, K. (2000). Time and medical education. *Annals of Internal Medicine, 132,* 25–28.

Mackway-Jones, K., & Walker, M. (1999). *Pocket guide to teaching for medical instructors.* London: BMJ Books.

Malone, M., & Jackson, T. (1993). Educational characteristics of an ambulatory morning report. *Journal of General Internal Medicine, 8,* 512–514.

Mcdonagh, J. (1997). Rheumatology outpatient training: Time for a re-think? *Annals of Rheumatic Diseases, 56,* 701–704.

McKeachie, W. (1986). *A guidebook for the beginning college teacher* (8th ed.). Lexington, MA: Heath & Company.

Morrell, D. (1981). Sampling medical records. In J. Cormack, M. Marinker, & D. Morrell (Eds.), *Teaching general practice.* London: Kluwer Medical.

Norman, G., Barrows, H., Gliva, G., & Woodward, C. (1985). Simulated patients. In V. Neufeld & G. Norman (Eds.), *Assessing clinical competence.* New York: Springer Publishing.

Norman, G., Davis, D., Painvin, A., Lindsay, E., Rath, D., & Ragbeer, M. (1989). Comprehensive assessment of clinical competence of family/general practitioners using multiple measures. In *Research in medical education: 1989: Proceedings of the Twenty-eighth Annual Conference.* Washington, DC: Association of American Medical Colleges.

Paccione, G., Cohen, E., & Schwartz, C. (1989). From forms to focus: A new teaching model in ambulatory medicine. *Annals of Internal Medicine, 149,* 2407–2411.

Premi, J. (1991). An assessment of 15 years experience in using videotape in a family practice residency. *Academic Medicine, 66,* 56–57.

Reinhart, M., & Keef, C. (1990). Individual differences in continuing professional competence: The sample case of emergency medicine physicians. In S. Willis & S. Dubin (Eds.), *Contemporary approaches to maintaining professional competence.* San Francisco: Jossey-Bass.

Schwenk, T., & Whitman, N. (1993). *Residents as teachers: A guide to educational practice.* Salt Lake City: University of Utah School of Medicine.

Siegel, S. (1998). Self-directed learning: Using patient simulations. *Education for General Practice, 9,* s502–503.

Shaughnessy, A., Slawson, D., & Becker, L. (1998). Clinical jazz: Harmonizing clinical experience and evidence-based medicine. *Journal of Family Practice, 47,* 425–428.

Smith, C., & Irby, D. (1997). The roles of experience and reflection in ambulatory care education. *Academic Medicine, 72,* 32–35.

Solomon, D., Reinhart, M., Bridgham, R., Munger, B., & Starnaman, S. (1990). An assessment of an oral examination format for evaluating clinical competence in emergency medicine. *Academic Medicine Supplement, 65,* S43–45.

Speedie, S., Pacala, J., & Vercellotti, G. (2001). Personal digital assistant support for outpatient clinical clerkships: Mobile computing for medical education. *Journal of the American Medical Informatics Association, Suppl. S,* 632–636.

Steinert, Y. (1993). Twelve tips for using role-play in clinical teaching. *Medical Teacher, 15,* 283–291.

Tiberius, R. (1995). *Small group teaching: A trouble-shooting guide.* Toronto: OISE Press/ Ontario Institute for Studies in Education.

Tugwell, P., & Dok, C. (1985). Medical record review. In V. Neufeld & G. Norman (Eds.), *Assessing clinical competence.* New York: Springer.

Vinson, D., Paden, C., Devera-Sales, A., Marshall, B., & Waters, C. (1997). Teaching medical students in community-based practices: A national survey of generalist physicians. *Journal of Family Practice, 6,* 487–494.

Westberg, J., & Jason, H. (1994). *Teaching creatively with video.* New York: Springer Publishing.

Westberg, J., & Jason, H. (1996). *Fostering learning in small groups.* New York: Springer Publishing.

Woolliscroft, J. O., Calhoun, J., Beauchamp, C., Wolf, F., & Maxim, B. (1984). Evaluating the medical history: Observation versus write-up review. *Journal of Medical Education, 59,* 19–23.

Wright, V., & Helliwell, P. (1991). Educating doctors about rheumatology. *Annals of Rheumatic Diseases, 50,* 439–444.

—5—

Special Learning Situations

It has been a year now since medical students and residents have been coming to Dr. Smith's group practice. Overall it has been a positive experience for the staff, and the evaluations from the trainees of their time spent have been favorable and appreciative. The patients have responded positively, and the medical teachers are becoming more comfortable with the ambulatory care teaching strategies. As one of Dr. Smith's colleagues said: "When a motivated student encounters an enthusiastic teacher in a conducive environment, learning seems easy."

As Dr. Smith and his associates have also discovered, however, office procedures do not always run smoothly. The doctors have had some trainees who have created challenges in the office by interfering with the learning of other students or by frustrating both the teachers and the rest of the office staff. The doctors decided to devote their next evening session to a review of the difficult learning situations they have had in the office during the last year, and to try to develop some mechanisms for dealing with the problems in the future. To assist them, they invited the director of the department of medical education at the local faculty of medicine to act as a resource. A summary of their deliberations about some general principles follows.

1. Begin to deal with a problem situation as soon as it is recognized as such (McGraw & Verma, 2001).
2. Document examples of the problem so that you can be specific with trainees when discussing the issue. Keep a file of these examples

as they occur. You will not remember many of them when trainees challenge you and ask for specific examples of the problem.

3. Meet with trainees and make them aware of your concerns. Obtain their viewpoint and set up a jointly agreed-upon plan for dealing with the problem (Shapiro, Prislin, Larsen, & Lenahan, 1987).

4. Each situation is the result of a dynamic between three factors: the learner, the teacher, and the learning environment. Approach the solution by dealing with each of these factors.

5. Some problems are related to the trainee's personality. A teacher is not a psychotherapist and is not expected to diagnose or treat well-established traits. If a personality issue seems to be playing a role in the problem, however, you can at least make the learner aware of the situation. The dean's office or program director can then help the student, if more in-depth treatment is a solution. In the meantime, there are some initial strategies to use in your office that will help you deal with certain personality types when they interfere with learning.

6. Arrange a follow-up meeting with the trainee to monitor progress with the plan of action.

7. Some of these problems may be preventable. By understanding and applying principles of learning to your teaching, you may prevent some of these problems from occurring.

8. You will rarely be able to resolve for the learner any of these problem situations completely. In ambulatory care teaching, your encounter with the student will, in most cases, be only a small fraction of his training time. You can start the process, however, by helping the learner realize the problem and by setting up an initial plan to work on while he is with you.

9. If you notice a recurring problem in students rotating through your ambulatory care teaching center, consult with the dean's office or program director. There may be some behavior that the students are learning in their basic training, an unbeknownst consequence of the curriculum.

SUMMARY OF SPECIAL LEARNING SITUATIONS

This is the list of situations with learners that Dr. Smith's group was able to compile based on their previous encounters with students.

Clinical Learning Situations

- Clinical judgment difficulty
- Poor knowledge base
- Slow worker
- Premature closure of inquiry

Patient-Related Situations

- Ethnic, racial, or gender prejudices
- Avoidance of difficult patients
- Inappropriate grooming or dress

Teacher-Learner Interaction

- Argumentative with teaching staff
- Defensive about errors or weaknesses
- Disruptive of group learning
- Nonresponder to questions
- Noncommittal to management plans
- Sycophantic toward staff

Personal Issues

- Overconfident as doctor
- Overinvolved with patients
- Overloaded with commitments
- Shy with colleagues and staff
- Lazy at work
- Psychiatric problems
- Lack of self-direction in learning
- Lying to teaching staff
- Substance abuse

Of course, none of these situations is exclusive to ambulatory care teaching. But because of the nature of ambulatory care teaching, with its intensive one-to-one teaching, these problems are often more apparent.

They may have more impact on an office routine than in a hospital ward, where the team structure will help to diffuse the problem and not let it affect patient care. The learner may be sheltered by the team, which can hinder the problem from becoming evident. Your office is an ideal setting to begin the process of change.

Let us now examine each of these special situations; examine the dynamic between the learner, teacher, and the environment; and describe some strategies that we have used to help teachers and learners deal with problems.

CLINICAL LEARNING SITUATIONS

Clinical Judgment Difficulty

Issue: Inability to make appropriate, logical, or correct decisions based on the evidence.

Presentation: In clinical decision making, knowledge and experience help the physician choose an appropriate route of action. Learners with poor judgment tend to draw the wrong conclusion based on the available data. Their diagnostic choices do not follow from the clinical information. Management plans are not sensible. Word selection or approach to patients may be unsuitable.

Example: A final-year medical student is assigned to your office once a week throughout the first term. Her fund of medical knowledge is fairly good, as are her history-taking skills. On several occasions, however, when the available data pointed to a major illness, she diagnosed a less serious condition. At other times, she has not asked for help when she needed it. Her interpretation of laboratory results was not correct; thus, her recommendations based on those test results often did not follow logically. Yet, at other times she dwelled inappropriately on several worst case scenarios, upsetting her patients in the process.

Considerations: When you encounter a learner with poor judgment, the following may be factors.

- A poor knowledge base may affect the learner's ability to draw appropriate conclusions.

- Lack of clinical experience may lead the learner down the wrong track.
- Anxiety, either from a personal problem or related to pressure from the teacher or the office setting (e.g., demanding teacher, busy office), can interfere with judgment. (Anxiety interferes with concentration, causing the learner to miss cues or hurry to an incorrect diagnosis.)
- Overwork and fatigue cloud judgment by impairing concentration and by limiting patience for detail.
- Some learners cannot set priorities, are disorganized in their thinking, and cannot distinguish serious from trivial conditions.

Management: The following are helpful in managing these difficulties.

- Discuss concerns with the learner and provide specific examples of the behavior.
- If there is poor knowledge, set a learning plan.
- If it seems that the main problem is a lack of experience, take a little more time to discuss each case as it occurs, and highlight clues in the clinical presentation that lead to the diagnosis.
- Explore the trainee's personal anxieties, or ask about difficulties in working in the current setting.
- If fatigue is an issue, review the learner's work or call schedule, and discuss it with the program director. Sometimes, what the trainee really needs is a vacation.
- Trainees can learn about the weighing of clinical evidence by learning about the concepts of prevalence and probabilities. They should be asked to rank common disorders first when presenting a differential diagnosis.
- For assisting trainees with the weighing of clinical evidence, the use of chart stimulated recall is the ideal strategy to further assess their clinical judgment and to provide suggestions for change.

Poor Knowledge Base

Issue: Insufficient or poor knowledge of the content of medicine, which should have been obtained before the current level of training.

Presentation: Learner is consistently unable to explain standard medical concepts, underlying pathophysiology, or differential diagnosis. Sometimes, the learner cannot elucidate a plan of investigation or has difficulty in outlining options for treatment. The student may also have an isolated gap in his knowledge base.

Example: One of your medical students has completed 2 weeks of a 4-week ambulatory medical rotation. The teaching staff comments that, despite "trying hard" and using seemingly reasonable judgment, there are just times when the student does not know the tests to order and cannot seem to explain underlying reasons for his diagnostic choices. In addition, although he knows which drugs to order, he makes errors in prescribing drugs.

Considerations: When you encounter this problem, the following may be factors.

- The learner may not have learned the required material during medical school. It may have been poorly taught or skipped altogether. Poor learning habits may have interfered with retaining the information (Quirk, 1994).
- Family or personal problems may have taken the student away from school or not allowed her to study.
- Social activities or extracurricular school activities may have interfered with reading time.
- The learner may have poor organization skills, learning enough to pass examinations but not enough to flourish in the clinical setting.
- Sometimes the learner has the knowledge, but the teacher is not providing clear questions, or may be quite demanding or overly critical.
- The learner may be shy and reluctant to demonstrate actual knowledge.

Management: The following are helpful in managing these difficulties.

- Check the learner's past evaluations to identify previous weaknesses in knowledge. An informal conversation with a previous supervisor may be helpful.
- Meet with the learner and explore the possibility of personal or emotional conflicts that may have interfered with learning. If these exist, refer the learner to the appropriate dean's office to identify opportunities for help.

- Set up a learning plan with the student to help fill in some of the gaps of knowledge during the ambulatory rotation. The student should be free to choose a preferred learning method, be it books, journals, websites, audiotapes, update courses, etc. The teacher should provide suggestions for resources, such as conferences and courses. There should be regular meetings to assess progress with the learning plan and to modify it as necessary.
- Encourage the learner to read about a specific problem when it arises (i.e., in response to cases seen in the office). Some students may benefit from a problem-oriented textbook.
- If, in discussion, it becomes apparent that the learner knows more than has been evident and has been shy to speak up, refer to a later section for suggestions.

Slow Worker

Issue: This learner seems to spend excessive time with patients and is constantly behind schedule.

Presentation: You will recognize this situation when the two of you are always the last ones to leave each day. The student spends a great deal of time with each patient, not necessarily constructively. Before you even realize it, he is way behind in the schedule of patients. Patients are often seen more than an hour late.

Example: A final-year medical student is working in your office this month. Each night you leave the office later and later. You always seem to be waiting for the student to finish his last patient. When you observe him at work, he somehow manages to make a short visit into a long one. There are great delays between seeing patients, and you cannot figure out what he is doing. Everything takes twice as long than it does with any other final-year student that you have had in your office.

Considerations: When you encounter this problem, the following may be factors.

- Each case is usually multifactorial, and each needs to be handled individually. Every part of the patient-doctor interaction can be a partial source of delay. The student may be unable to do a focused history and physical examination, or may talk at great length. Lack of confidence or lack of experience can interfere with decision making and thus slow each step along the way. Lack of knowledge of office routines will cause the student to spend extra time between patients making arrangements for tests, consultations, and so on.

- Some students may be booked with too many patients for their level of training.
- The teaching physician may take too much time between cases discussing the management and further delay the student.

Management: The following are helpful in managing these difficulties.

- Try to determine with the student where the delays seem to be occurring. If available, a videotape review of patient sessions will help to pinpoint the areas of slowdown.
- Remember, the problem is usually multifactorial, and each problem needs to be handled on an individual basis, as follows:

  - *Lack of knowledge of office routines:* Ask an office nurse or secretary to give special assistance to the student to arrange laboratory tests, give injections, or call consultants.
  - *Lengthy explanations:* Learners often equate time spent with quality of the interaction. They need to be taught that a brief but clear explanation to the patient, leaving opportunity for questions, is even better than a long-winded conclusion to the encounter. The best method would be to demonstrate this using role modeling or role play.
  - *Detailed history taking:* Each specialty has its own version of a focused history, and trainees, especially in the junior years, need to be guided in asking the appropriate questions for a history in your type of ambulatory setting.
  - *Lack of confidence or experience:* The trainee cannot move on from step to step in the patient encounter because of fear of making an error or of missing something. Experience will eventually help this learner, but, in the meantime, you can demonstrate from your own experience how the concepts of prevalence and likelihood allow you to move from step to step in the patient encounter.

- Try booking fewer patients with the trainee, and then increase the number booked per session as the learner shows that he can handle them in the allotted time.

- When appropriate, limit discussion time between patients to the essentials for patient care, and then refer to chapter 4 for additional ideas on other times for teaching.

Premature Closure of Inquiry

Issue: The learner narrows down the diagnosis prematurely.

Presentation: There are two situations in which this issue is evident. First, when a learner takes a history from a patient, the series of questions will narrow quickly and exclude a wider range of diagnoses. Similarly, in discussion of differential diagnosis, one dominant option will be presented by the learner with little consideration of a wider differential diagnosis.

Example: You are observing a resident via a video camera. She has been interviewing an elderly patient who presents with weakness. After a few general questions, the resident begins to ask a series of closed questions that focus on confirming a suspicion of depression. Questions are asked in a manner to make the answers fit the diagnosis. There are no other questions asked that might help to rule out other possible causes of weakness.

Considerations: Premature closure can result from any of the following.

- There may be a weakness in the trainee's interviewing skills. He may not have learned the concept of listening to the patient, especially if his medical school does not have an interviewing skills course.
- Some students use closed questions because they have been taught to take a medical history by following a series of defined questions to narrow down the diagnosis to one possibility. Students learn that the object of the game is to find a single diagnosis, and the teacher may unwittingly reinforce this need to find the diagnosis.
- The student may lack knowledge, not know the appropriate questions to ask, and focus on an area that he knows for greater comfort.
- The student may be pressed for time because of a heavy load of patients and is anxious to get to a diagnosis quickly. Because of inexperience, he thinks that a series of short, quick questions will get him more rapidly to the diagnosis.

- Sometimes the student may be overconfident or insecure, and needs to bolster his self-esteem with quick success.

Management: The following are helpful in managing these difficulties.

- If you have videotape or audiotape, you should show him an example of premature closure. Otherwise, if you have observed an encounter, repeat for the student the approximate sequence of questions. Then, using role play, try to have the student do the interview again, taking more time to listen to the patient or using open-ended questions that expand the range of diagnostic possibilities. This can be repeated once a week until the learner has a better idea of the problem.
- The learner can practice the use of open-ended questions in general, for example, as follows:

Teacher: A patient presents with abdominal pain. Try to list for me several questions that you might ask without specifically asking about the pain.

Student: "Can you tell me more about it?" "Can you tell me what led up to it?" "What is concerning you about it?"

- If the problem is limited knowledge blocking the exploration of other options, refer to the previous section for a method to improve knowledge.
- If you conclude that the student is overconfident, see a later section for help.
- Ensure that the trainee is not booked with too many patients for his level of training.
- Use every opportunity to ask the student the widest possible range of differential diagnoses. Consider as well that in ambulatory care there is often no certain conclusion on diagnosis reached at many visits.
- Remember that this is another type of problem for which stimulated chart review can be used effectively. As the learner talks aloud about the interview, draw his attention to points at which he seemed to come to an early conclusion about the diagnosis and ask him to expand his range of possibilities. Then point out how this new range of possible diagnoses will change the sequence of questions to follow.

PATIENT-RELATED SITUATIONS

Ethnic, Racial, or Gender Prejudices

Issue: The learner has a belief, sometimes religious in origin, or a particular bias that affects decision making, patient counseling, or the doctor-patient interaction.

Presentation: Belief or bias can interfere with history taking and patient management. There may be biases that are based on family background or other important life experiences that are a major issue for the learner.

Example: Staff has noticed that a resident has difficulty in dealing with gay patients. He is obviously very uncomfortable in the interview. He has difficulty asking about sexual orientation. He is fearful of HIV disease and the risk of patient contact for health care workers. He offers little sympathy to such patients.

Considerations: Biases or prejudices are learned attitudes or behaviors that develop as the child grows. These beliefs are acquired from parents, relatives, friends, and school interactions.

Management: In ambulatory care, the teacher's role is to identify learner biases that impact on patient care, not to try to change long-standing beliefs. Meet with the trainee, and provide specific examples. Discuss with the trainee his ethical responsibility toward the patient, and develop strategies to ensure that the bias does not interfere with that patient's care.

Avoidance of Difficult Patients

Issue: This learner avoids contact with specific groups of patients with which she does not enjoy working or which she has trouble handling.

Presentation: There are certain groups of patients that learners will often avoid seeing if possible. These include the elderly, people of low socioeconomic status, the unkempt, the difficult historians, and the disabled. Also, difficult patients, such as dependent, demanding, or hostile ones, are by-passed. The student creates every imaginable reason why he cannot see the patient (e.g., I'm way behind, this is John's patient, etc.). If the trainee has to see the patient, she spends the least amount of time possible.

Example: A resident in the ambulatory clinic this month has been rude to some of the young teenage mothers. She often makes derogatory comments about people who lack formal education. Several times she has left these mothers waiting for long periods while she tended to nonurgent matters in the inpatient unit. When her behavior with them was observed, she was seen to be abrupt and impatient and not attentive to their concerns about problems with their children.

Considerations: Most medical learners have middle-class norms that can interfere with their interactions with other different groups (Klein, Najman, Kohrman, & Munro, 1982).

Difficult patients evoke emotional negative reactions in doctors that often go unrecognized. The mere sight of the patient's name on the day list can ruin an afternoon. An office visit or telephone call can leave the doctor frustrated. Doctors deny these feelings of "hatred" toward these patients and then let these feelings affect future interactions (Groves, 1978).

Management: Use of patient profiles for trainees will help document avoidance of a particular group of patients.

To help trainees deal with difficult patients, you must alert them to the emotional reaction these patients are causing. When discussing such a patient in case review or chart review sessions, ask trainees about the feelings that were provoked by that patient. Help them to realize that their reaction is not unique and that it is proper for them to acknowledge these emotions. Reference to literature describing doctors' common reactions to these types of patients will help them accept these feelings as normal (Anstett, 1980; Groves, 1978; Klein et al., 1982). You can then develop a strategy with the trainee to deal with this patient in the future (Herbert & Grams, 1986). This should include the following:

- Help the patient to clearly identify the problem to be addressed (e.g., Which problem should we talk about today?).
- Acknowledge the patient's feelings directly (e.g., You sound angry today).
- Find the source of the feeling (e.g., Is there anyone in particular at whom you are angry?).

- Develop an explicit management plan involving the patient, including a channeling of the trainee's emotional energy in a positive manner.

If time permits, use of role play to practice some of these strategies can be very beneficial. Both teacher and trainee can play the role of the difficult patient, with the other practicing strategies.

Inappropriate Grooming or Dress

Issue: Conflicts in learning may arise when the student's physical appearance, dress, or other matters of image distract from the educational experience.

Presentation: The student may choose to dress in simpler clothing (e.g., blue jeans or T-shirt, which the teaching staff may consider inappropriate for this setting). Sometimes students come to ambulatory settings in their blood-covered scrub outfits rather than changing to their regular clothes. Problems of hygiene sometimes are apparent, such as hair, breath, or clean clothes. Teaching staff often comment on the seductively dressed female learner or the male learner who spends more on clothes than all the staff. Typically, the short, young-looking learner will constantly hear from patients that "you look too young to be a doctor." This may inhibit the establishment of a doctor-patient relationship and affect learning.

Example: There is a medical student working once a week in the outpatient department whose personal hygiene leaves much to be desired. His hair is unkempt, he wears the same old white shirt with black jeans, and his shirt is always hanging out from his pants. Despite a pleasant demeanor, he resembles the teenage volunteer worker at the reception desk.

Considerations: When issues of inappropriate dress arise, consider the following.

- Often the learner is not aware that his dress or appearance is a problem.
- The dress pattern may be the one he has always used and perhaps cannot afford others.
- Dress is often a personal statement of belonging to a certain group or an anti-establishment comment.

- Outrageous dress may be a method of calling attention to oneself. The one who wears old clothes or is unkempt and dirty may have little self-respect and thus feel no need to dress well.

Management: The following are helpful when dealing with these difficulties.

- Students need to be alerted to the problem, either with direct comment or through a videotape session. Teachers should discuss with learners their own impression of their dress and its meaning to learners as well as its potential impact on patient care.
- Apply the principles of process learning in this case. The issues of dress and appearance are often set by how the physicians and office staff dress when they are on the job.
- It is often simplest to set minimum dress standards, after consultation with the learners' representatives.
- The young-looking student can often be encouraged to dress "older."

TEACHER-LEARNER INTERACTION

Argumentative with Teaching Staff

Issue: Discussions with the learner easily turn into battles and debates.

Presentation: This learner cannot carry on a discussion without getting into a debate or argument with the teaching staff. Even innocuous conversations about patients end up as a battle of words and wills.

Example: A senior resident working with you in the outpatient clinic is very knowledgeable and a hard worker. She has a tendency, however, to dispute the management of most patients with you. She can be quite stubborn. Her interpretations are not incorrect, but she will stretch a weak point to the limit. You once got into a shouting match with her about the need to admit a patient for investigation. She quarrels with the nurses about the completion of laboratory forms and the secretaries about missing charts.

Considerations: When you encounter this problem, the following may be factors.

- The learner may have some personal upset that is making her angry, and she is transferring this to the work setting. She may be angry or concerned about some policy or work matter that she has been unwilling to discuss and is acting out her anger. Some learners need to be independent and cannot submit to authority. This is frequently a carryover of adolescent behavior.
- The argumentativeness may actually be a defense mechanism. The individual may fear dependence because she really needs to be told what to do. She is expressing a conflict between her fears of dependence and needs of guidance.
- Some arguments stem from a clash in the personalities or work habits of teacher and trainee.

Management: The teacher should arrange a meeting with the learner. Begin by citing specific examples of argumentative behavior. Next, inquire about any personal problems affecting the learner, or any policies or personnel around the office that may be causing this behavior.

If a personality type is recognized, the teacher should try to respond as follows.

- Give the "rebelling adolescent" some more independence as long as his actions do not affect patient care.
- If there seems to be a fear of dependence, try to highlight for the student the positive learning benefits of careful guidance rather than viewing it as control.
- Kind understanding of the angry trainee may decrease her acting-out behavior.

After adjustments for the preceding, knowing and tolerating each other's obsessions may prevent disagreements.

This approach provides some immediate solutions during the ambulatory care time. If this is a persistent issue, however, it would be appropriate to refer the trainee to the dean's office for advice or professional help.

Defensive About Errors or Weaknesses

Issue: Persistent attempts to justify or excuse errors, weaknesses, or gaps in knowledge, each of which removes the problem beyond the learner's control.

Presentation: When you are criticizing the learner for a specific behavior, he will rationalize his actions. At the time for evaluation, each negative comment will be explained in detail, providing reason and circumstances that resulted in the behavior. Most often, such rationalizations blame circumstances, or even others, for the bad outcome.

Example: A junior resident has just completed a month on a surgical ambulatory experience. His teacher finds him deficient in physical examination skills, knowledge of therapeutics, and charting. The resident explains that no one ever observed him do a complete physical examination, only small segments; that the knowledge gap in therapeutics resulted because his reading plan was interrupted by a heavy call schedule as a result of other residents' holidays; and that he was booked too heavily and had many late-arriving patients so there was little time for charting.

Considerations: When you encounter this problem, the following may be factors.

- The defensive learner lacks skill in self-assessment or reflection.
- There may be psychosocial problems resulting in low self-esteem. Such a trainee may come from a rigid family and conservative education system where nothing but excellence is tolerated.
- The teacher may have been particularly critical with this learner, forcing him to be defensive.

Management: There is certainly little use in debating each excuse made by a defensive learner. A more constructive approach is the use of a learning contract. This approach improves the learner's self-assessment skills rather than making him respond to your comments.

Using the concepts of process learning, you can establish an environment to defuse defensive behavior by the following:

- Act in a collegial manner with learners, and thus set a comfortable scene for comments on performance.
- Involve learners in discussions with your colleagues on your own cases in which the natural give-and-take is to share information and provide comments on each other's performance. This will help students learn that continued learning throughout one's career is the norm and that learning is enhanced by comments from others.
- Refer more difficult concerns such as low self-esteem for further assessment.

Disruptive of Group Learning

Issue: This learner will interfere with group learning by displaying domination or showmanship.

Presentation: Short didactic presentation or case review are common teaching methods used in the ambulatory setting. This process can be disrupted by the presence of an individual who dominates the group by talking at length, whether a question has been asked or not. She may ask questions that may or may not be relevant to the situation. She may also disrupt the group with loud laughter or constant joking.

Example: The clinic holds a weekly seminar on management issues of problem cases. Since the arrival of a new first-year resident, the sessions have not met their objectives. In addition, the clinical clerks have begun to complain that they are not learning anything at the seminar and are wasting their time. It has been reported that the resident presents a case, interspersed with jokes, and then presents a lengthy monologue of her personal opinions on management. As the seminar leader continues to lead the discussion, she interrupts with more picayune questions or jumps into the discussion by answering any question put to the group by the leader.

Considerations: The dominant speaker may be an outgoing person by nature, may think that her point may have not been heard or appreciated, or may feel compelled to compete with others in the group (Tiberius, 1995).
   Others may have an excessive need for power or attention. Some of the showing off may even be to hide fear of being found out.

Management: Talk privately to the learner who dominates or disrupts the group. She is usually not aware of the issue. Channel the energy of this individual in a positive manner by giving her a definite leadership role in the session. She should be instructed to present cases and then lead the questioning instead of responding to questions. Often she will thrive in this role, and the disruptive element is eliminated (Mackway-Jones & Walker, 1999).

Nonresponder to Questions

Issue: Lack of spontaneous comments when directly spoken to in a one-to-one situation or in group discussion.

Presentation: This learner does little to enhance group discussions. In a one-to-one setting, the learner will provide you with simple, brief answers to your questions and rarely asks questions himself.

Example: A resident is one of the several house staff rotating through the Family Medicine service. In the daily chart review he presents his cases in a brief manner. Between patients, when there is case discussion, he will not spontaneously offer any comments. At the weekly seminar he does not join in the discussion with his colleagues.

Considerations: The trainee may be afraid to reveal his gaps in knowledge. The learner may also have much of the required information, but because of a shy personality or because of his cultural background, he does not speak much outside the learning situation either (Tiberius, 1995). The teacher may be impatient with such a student or fail to establish a supportive environment in which a learner may feel free to talk or find it permissible to make mistakes.

Management: The following are helpful when dealing with nonresponders.

- During a private conversation with the trainee, try to understand why he is reluctant to participate in discussions. Ask him how both of you might contribute to helping him overcome this inhibition.
- Apply the principles of adult learning. Set up with the learner a nonthreatening environment, encourage him to use his current reservoir of knowledge, and let him know whenever he does something right.
- Address questions to this trainee that are easy to answer and then follow up with more detailed questions to engage him in the conversation.
- Avoid questions that can be answered with yes or no; require a more complete response (Tiberius, 1995).
- Try to be especially patient and spend a little more time rephrasing questions as you guide the trainee to the teaching point.

Noncommittal to Management Plans

Issue: Learner is unable or unwilling to outline a management plan in clinical situations.

Presentation: The student sees a patient and performs an appropriate assessment. After presenting the history and physical, the student does not offer any thoughts on the differential diagnosis, nor will she suggest a suitable management plan.

Example: A final-year medical student is several months into a weekly longitudinal ambulatory medical experience. She sees her patients and completes a thorough history and physical in each case. After presenting the case to her supervisor, she awaits direction from the supervisor. In some cases, she offers a differential diagnosis but then asks the supervisor, "What should I do now?" Even when asked specifically what she would do, the student avoids providing an answer.

Considerations: When you encounter this problem, the following may be factors.

- The student may have inadequate knowledge of clinical management, despite adequate knowledge of the basics of patient assessment.
- The student may be unwilling to offer a possible management plan for fear of making a mistake and looking "bad."
- The teacher might have established the environment that, for example, the office is always hurried and that there is little time to fumble around with discussion of the management plan. Sometimes, the teacher tells the student what to do after each patient is presented, and thus the student is programmed to wait for directions. In addition, the teacher may have been critical of the student when she presented management plans and thus suppressed any willingness by the student to take a chance if she is not sure of the correct treatment, for fear of being put to shame.

Management: The following are helpful when dealing with these difficulties.

- In the earlier years of training, knowledge of the clinical management of the patient lags far behind the skills of patient assessment and knowledge of disease. Early on, students should be encouraged to develop knowledge in patient management. Tell them that such knowledge comes with the experience of seeing patients and reading related journals and texts.
- If the student still seems unwilling to offer suggested management plans, the teacher needs to further use the skills of inquiry to help

the student bring the patient's problems together and to explore the student's knowledge reservoir.
- Failing this approach, the student may lack knowledge. Use chart-stimulated recall with the learner to get at the deficiencies, and set up a learning plan.
- The teacher should also look at his own method of reviewing patients with the students and ensure that he is supportive of learning and not just getting through the patient list. It should be acceptable for a trainee to make mistakes, to fall behind a little as she struggles with questions, or to give the wrong answer as a normal part of learning.

Sycophantic Toward Staff

Issue: This is the learner who loves too much!

Presentation: The learner tends to be overly attentive to the staff and very flattering. There is constant regard for the talents and knowledge of the teacher and a fawning, ingratiating approach. Because of the learner's demeanor, you cannot bear much time teaching him and make the encounters as brief as possible or even avoid him if you can. There is serious interruption of the teacher-learner relationship.

Example: You are working with a family medicine resident in your hospital-based practice. This student is forever hanging on your every word. He is constantly all smiles. It is always, Dr. this . . . or Dr. that. . . . He tells you that your knowledge of medicine and clinical acumen is excellent, except he says it twice a day. You feel a need to "brush him aside" because he seems to be "all over you."

Considerations: When you encounter this problem, the following may be factors.

- These trainees may have a need to be liked or to be protected. They may have difficulty in dealing with authority and cope with this difficulty by being ingratiating.
- Sometimes, the trainee wants to share the authority's power by attaching to it.
- Others may be trying to hide a poor knowledge base or lack of technical skill with this flattering behavior.

Management: The most difficult thing is to resist the urge to tell this student to cut the nonsense and stop smiling all the time. This problem is an excellent example of how the relatively brief exposures that teachers have with students in the ambulatory setting make it difficult to deal with personality issues that can inhibit learning.

In this case, an acknowledgment of the compliment and a gentle statement that no further commendation is necessary may help you return to a more comfortable interaction with the student. If you have a longer period with the student, you may gradually explore his feelings about authority to get a better understanding of the individual and then eventually bring to his attention some of this behavior.

PERSONAL ISSUES

Overconfident as Doctor

Issue: The trainee attempts to function at a level that is inappropriately advanced for his stage of education.

Presentation: The trainee appears overconfident in his daily work. He tries to function as an experienced doctor beyond his years.

Example: A resident on the outpatient clinic rotation works quite rapidly, presenting his cases with assurance. He concludes with his most likely diagnosis and management plan, both of which may be far from the correct route. He attempts to perform procedures with which he has little experience. He resists considering other diagnoses.

Considerations: This behavior can be overcompensation or a defense mechanism for deficits that the learner is attempting to hide. There may be actual knowledge lack, poor technical skill, or other deficits that the student fears will be uncovered, and he uses this as a defense mechanism because of this fear.

Sometimes, the trainee has a narcissistic personality type. These individuals generally feel good about themselves, are self-centered, and are not empathic or understanding (Akhtar, 1989).

Alternatively, the teacher may be one who easily intimidates students with authority or belittles their knowledge. The learner may compensate for this with overconfident behavior.

Management: When encountering an overconfident trainee who does not have the knowledge he purports, one must monitor the learner carefully. Supervise his clinical performance by using case discussions, chart audits, or case reviews. Using the Socratic method, explore in detail his diagnostic plans. When more time is available, chart-stimulated recall will help both of you understand his problem-solving method. Gradually, he will become aware of his true level of performance.

If the student's knowledge and skill level seem adequate for his level of training, you are more likely dealing with a personality type. The simplest route is to use directive teaching to provide clear but firm examples to show to the learner that he is performing at his level of training but not higher. His energies can be directed toward further acquisition of knowledge and skills in his search for excellence. As a teacher, you do not have the knowledge, skill, or time to deal with the personality disorder.

Overinvolved with Patients

Issue: Excessive commitment and feelings of obligation to patients and work responsibilities.

Presentation: The patients and their problems become all consuming for the learner. Inordinate amounts of time are spent with patients. There is an emotional involvement with the patient that is more familial than that of a caring professional. There is a boundary problem, that is, an inability to separate and define the limits of his responsibility to his patients.

Example: A junior resident is in your practice for the month. She is always behind schedule with patients. She can easily spend 45 minutes following up a routine problem. You have had the opportunity to observe her in an interview. She becomes very engrossed in the patient's life details, beyond what is relevant to the current situation or problem. She seems to be constantly on the telephone organizing details for certain patients. She gave her home telephone number to some families if they needed assistance during the month.

Considerations: When you encounter this problem, the following may be factors.

• Certain students cannot define their role as physician and do not understand the delegation of work to other health workers.

- Some students equate total time spent with the patient with effective outcome rather than looking at the end result.
- Some individuals have a need to be wanted or depended on by patients.

Management: The following are helpful in dealing with overinvolvement.

- Demonstrate how the same ends could be achieved in shorter time spans by discussing cases in which the trainee seemed to be overinvolved. You could use the role-play strategy best in this scenario.
- During case discussion with the learner, discuss how the various personnel available in the office or health care system can help him achieve the goals he has in mind for the patient.
- If you have a sense that a personal need is being met with this behavior, you could use time in case review, when the teaching is less focused on the one individual, to teach about the need to separate one's professional self from the personal.

Overloaded with Commitments

Issue: Learner is preoccupied, or involved in work or other activities that interfere with function or learning on the job.

Presentation: This behavior usually manifests as a general decrease in work performance. There may be evidence of fatigue or low energy. Concentration on work is a problem, and the details of work are not completed in a satisfactory manner. At first, the trainee may be regarded as lazy or unmotivated. The problem, however, may be related to overwork (i.e., too many patients to see, too many rounds to present, involvement in hospital committees, etc.). Moonlighting is another cause of fatigue and disinterest. Outside interests may compete for his time and attention.

Example: A student doing an elective arrives late most mornings to the clinic and looks quite tired. She has called in to cancel some appointments without adequate explanation, and several times has left early before all the patients were reviewed. She tells you that she has to commute a long distance each day because her partner is working in the next town. She is actively involved in a dance group that meets several nights a week. She works for a housecall service on weekends.

Considerations: When you encounter this problem, the following may be factors.

- These learners are unable to set priorities and manage their time. They resent the impact of medical life on their outside activities and try to carry a full load of extracurricular activities.
- They may have to moonlight to pay off debts or to obtain extra money for discretionary spending.
- Teachers sometimes load up learners with additional patients and rounds of assignments, without knowing their other responsibilities.

Management: Meet with the trainee and outline the problem to her, providing specific examples that you have kept on file. After getting her perspective on the issue, ask her to prepare for the next day a schedule listing all the previous week's activities. This should include work, educational programs, extracurricular activities, travel time, and pleasure activities. She should account for all the waking hours of the day, including weekends. At the next session, review this with her, and discuss its impact on her life and work. There will be a need to discuss, in general, her life priorities, and ways to manage time effectively to achieve her goals. She could be referred to appropriate books and articles on time management. In this review also check to see whether she has been assigned an excessive load of patient or educational tasks.

This scenario is a good situation for process learning and role modeling. It is hoped that you and your colleagues have their time management skills in order. In ambulatory care settings, the trainee is, in a sense, living with you and your colleagues. (In some smaller towns, trainees often do live in the home of one of the doctors while on rotation from the medical school.) By being part of a well-managed office and seeing your own personal life, the trainee will learn how to arrange her own time successfully.

Shy with Colleagues and Staff

Issue: The shy student is reserved, avoids familiarity or contact with colleagues, and tends to work unobtrusively.

Presentation: This learner is difficult to get to know. She is quiet and rarely engages in random conversation. She volunteers little of herself and her personal life. She avoids the teaching staff and may be known as a loner.

Example: A second-year resident has been coming to the ambulatory clinics twice a week for 3 months. All the staff have commented that she is very shy. She seldom says hello to anyone at the clinic. Little is known of her personal life, and she leaves quickly at the end of work. She does not engage in the usual banter among staff in the clinic and is often described as cold. She rarely makes eye contact when talking to her supervisor. On reviewing her residency file, you find that other evaluations have commented on this shyness. When she is dealing with patients, however, she is quite outgoing, warm, and conversant.

Considerations: When you encounter this problem, the following may be factors.

- The shy learner may represent a personality type who has always been that way.
- Another type of character is the one who is anxious, often embarrassed, and inhibited. This learner is ruled by anxiety and is fearful of speaking out or having weaknesses discovered, whether real or not.
- The trainee may interact according to culture or family traditions.
- Sometimes, the teaching staff may be so formal and businesslike themselves that teachers and learners do not mix.

Management: The following are helpful when dealing with these difficulties.

- This is another opportunity for process learning. The teaching staff should try to engage the student in conversation, and should make it more obvious that it is acceptable to be friendly and open and that the teachers have a personal interest in the student. In a meeting with the student, the teacher should express the comments of the staff, explore the student's feelings about interactions with the teachers, and agree that everyone will make more of an effort to be supportive.
- If a significant personality problem seems to be interfering with patient care and the learner's future potential as a doctor, the possibilities for change through psychotherapy should be discussed with the trainee, perhaps through the dean's office.

Lazy at Work

Issue: Lack of enthusiasm and energy for learning and work-related responsibilities.

Presentation: The trainee shows overall lack of interest in educational activities. He does the bare minimum of work required in the office when booked with patients or in other practice activities such as hospital visits and on-call coverage.

Example: A clinical clerk is completing a 4-week experience in the ear, nose, and throat outpatient setting. He spends a great deal of time sitting in a lounge, waiting to be told about patients to be seen. He sees two or three patients per session when the others see five or six. He quickly reviews his cases with the clinic physician and leaves the hospital. He demonstrates little excitement about work or his patients. His presentation for rounds was inadequate for his level of training.

Considerations: When you encounter this problem, the following may be factors.

- This may be a general personality type, demonstrating low energy and low activity.
- Otherwise, this may be considered an issue of motivation. Motivation is one's willingness to exert a high level of effort to attain a goal. It is dependent on one's ability to satisfy some individual need (Robbins & Stuart-Kotze, 1990). It is the end result of the interaction between the individual and the situation. The trainee will weigh all the many conflicting demands and choose, either consciously or subconsciously, to work hard or not. Usually, basic requirements such as sleep and hunger must be satisfied before higher-order ones such as social needs, self-esteem, or personal learning interests (Maslow, 1954). A hardworking trainee may skip an excellent seminar related to his particular interest because he is too tired. Conversely, a normally lethargic trainee, a computer whiz, meets with the business manager every week to learn about the office computer system.
- The teacher's expectation may be too high, demanding each student to be as obsessive and hardworking as he is.
- In some circumstances, the work load may be excessive, and scheduling is inappropriate for the level of training.

Management: The following are helpful when dealing with laziness.

- Discuss the teacher's expectations for work load and educational activities with the trainee and ensure that the objectives for the ambulatory care rotation are clear with the trainee.

- Try to learn factors from the trainee that may be influencing his motivation. Help the trainee look at the factors affecting personal needs versus demands of the situation. It is a matter of being able to answer the question "Do I work hard right now?" If not, why not? Ensure that the basic needs for sleep and food are being met, and move on from there.
- Review the trainee's learning plan. Discuss his impressions of the work setting (i.e., his level of anxiety or sense of belonging).
- Ask about his personal life to see if there is any impact on his work. Try to adjust the variables so that "yes" is the answer to the work effort question.

Psychiatric Problems

Issue: Apparent behavioral, learning, or work problems are secondary to a more specific psychiatric diagnosis.

Presentation: The student's overall performance is poor, or perhaps his knowledge level is inferior to that of others. Sometimes the student appears to be uninvolved or lazy. When the problem is assessed, it becomes apparent that the underlying issue is a psychological problem interfering with performance.

Example: An clinical clerk is on the Internal Medicine ambulatory service. The staff has noticed that her knowledge of the content of medicine is poor. She is disorganized and accomplishes little work compared with her colleagues. She seems to be unenthusiastic and uninvolved. She is not up to date on her patients and their problems, and she shows little energy for work. In a meeting with her, the teacher learns that she is depressed. A planned marriage was broken off by her fiancé. Her father had died a year previously, and she has had to care for her mother, who is also quite depressed. She missed many classes after her father died and knew of huge gaps in her knowledge.

Considerations: Any psychiatric problem can interfere with work performance or learning. Before the work or knowledge can be improved, the underlying problem has to be treated. Often it is difficult for a physician to admit to an emotional problem because she wants to appear to be functioning well in front of teachers, colleagues, and friends.

The learning environment may contribute to the development of psychological problems. The student may be isolated in the work setting with little support from his peers. It may be a very competitive atmosphere that places unnecessary pressure on the student. As well, there may be unusually high expectations placed on the learner, which further increases stress levels.

Management: Teacher and trainee should meet to discuss the work problem and introduce the possibility of an emotional problem interfering with work. The teacher is not there to make a diagnosis but to alert the trainee to what might be occurring.

Together with the dean's office or the program director, the trainee can arrange psychiatric consultation outside the setting where the student is working so that the treatment remains fully confidential. Then, set up a learning plan to help fill in the gaps in knowledge and improve clinical areas of performance. Set up a schedule for regular performance reviews. If necessary, provide time off work for treatment of the psychiatric problem.

Lack of Self-Direction in Learning

Issue: The learner is unable to change behavior without specific external guidance.

Presentation: In the typical learning situations, this student depends on the teacher to be a primary source of information and adviser. He will, generally, not be willing or able to seek out, independently, sources of new material or people with whom to consult. These are the learners who want to be "spoon fed" or have everything "given to them on a silver platter." When given feedback, the learner will ask for detailed instruction on how to change the identified problem.

Example: You are working this month with a student who is interested in ophthalmology as a career. She attends the offices of all the ophthalmologists on a rotating basis each day. Each of the staff doctors has commented that she asks a lot of detailed questions about the various cases. When directed to read a particular item in response to a question, she never reports or comments that she may have done just that. In addition, she does not seem to read on her own initiative. She was unable to describe to the chief, who organized her elective, what she wanted to get out of her time in the department.

Considerations: Most humans seem to be born with an innate ability and interest in learning. Picture the young infant who is constantly exploring and learning at an incredible rate. Why, then, do we see so many mature learners arriving at our ambulatory teaching center waiting to be taught rather than eager to explore and learn? It is speculated that traditional school systems undermine this natural drive to learn. As the young child enters the traditional school system, what to learn is specifically defined, and most of the material is handed by the teacher to the student. Learning is geared to the lowest common denominator in most schools. This continues throughout precollege education and is reinforced by the well-defined curricula of most undergraduate schools. Even in medical schools, notes are handed out by instructors, then memorized and regurgitated by students. The student no longer knows how to learn on his own (Postman & Weingartner, 1969).

Management: The following are helpful in dealing with lack of self-direction.

- The student needs to be guided to use the skills of self-learning.
- Use learning plans, as described earlier in this book.
- In one-to-one office teaching, the teacher should help the student find out the answer to his questions. Discuss with the student where he might find the answers. Establish a time for the student to report back to the teacher on the method of finding the answer and a summary of the information obtained.

Lying to Teaching Staff

Issue: Learner shows a persistent tendency to create misleading impressions or to overtly deceive staff or patients.

Presentation: In its outright form, the learner is dishonest and is discovered. Often, it is a much more subtle issue that is not so black and white. The learner's behavior may be such that she acts to create an impression that may be far different from the one that exists. She may not be purposefully deceitful, but may stretch or bend the reality. Others may be described as more devious or crafty in their dealings or reasoning.

Example: A third-year medical student is doing a longitudinal elective in the ambulatory surgery clinic each week. Several times she stated that she had completed certain parts of the physical examination; however, because of obvious physical findings not reported, it had evidently not been done. The clinic manager could not trace a certain long-distance call made each week from the office to the same number. She denied making these calls until told that the clinic manager called the number and the party identified the medical student as the caller. In addition, one of the nurses saw her in the local shopping mall at lunch on a day she called in sick.

Considerations: One route to understanding the person who lies is to look at possible motivating factors. The lying may be serving a particular purpose, or it may be an easy way out—all factors that make the lying acceptable to the individual. Also examine the lack of guilt; the person has not developed a sense of values and thus has a selfish attitude of "serve yourself." There is little empathy and a "who cares?" approach.

At times, both teachers and educational institutions place incredible demands on their students. Sometimes, they find that they need to use deceit to survive. In addition, the perception that one cannot make a mistake, one must know everything, or one cannot ask for help—set up by teachers—causes learners to be dishonest.

Management: When caught, learners must be informed of the lie or dishonest act by their supervisor. They should be expected to make amends for any material loss. There may be extenuating circumstances to explain the dishonesty; otherwise students and teachers need to take time to discuss circumstances that may lead to such behavior. In light of such behavior, teaching staff need to look at the environment created to see if they are providing one that is open to honesty and positive criticism.

Substance Abuse

Issue: The use and abuse of both legal and illegal substances for nontherapeutic purposes by the learner.

Presentation: The learner may exhibit some of the classic manifestations of substance abuse: irritability, tremors, excessive absence from work, decrease in work performance, smells of alcohol, or even accidental overdose. The commonest addictions are those in the general community—alcohol, marijuana, hashish, cocaine, or benzodiazepines.

Example: A senior resident has missed at least two clinics per week during the last month. He usually calls at about 9:00 a.m., saying he is not feeling well and cannot come to work. In addition, when on call several times, he has not answered his pager. When he is at work, he appears energized and excitable with a somewhat bad temper. There have also been reports of large amounts of samples of lorazepam missing from the storage closet.

Considerations: Students at all levels of training are subjected to high stress, fatigue, high expectations, fear of failure, and easy access to legal drugs that could be abused.

Management: The learner must be confronted immediately with the suspicion of drug abuse. Then, refer the student to the dean's office or program director.

The health of the learner must be established as a priority. There should be an understanding that, if corrected, training will continue. Appropriate time off should be made available for treatment, whether it is a certain time each week or an extended leave of weeks or months.

Treatment is best provided in a facility away from the local clinic or hospital to ensure confidentiality. Referral via a local medical association or a resident association "hotline" will ensure trust and confidentiality.

REFERENCES

Akhtar, S. (1989). Narcissistic personality disorder. *Psychiatric Clinics of North America, 12*, 505–529.

Anstett, R. (1980). The difficult patient and the physician-patient relationship. *Journal of Family Practice, 11*, 281–286.

Groves, J. (1978). Taking care of the hateful patient. *New England Journal of Medicine, 298*, 883–887.

Herbert, C., & Grams, G. (1986). Working with the difficult patient: An approach for family physicians. *Canadian Family Physician, 32*, 1899–1905.

Klein, D., Najman, J., Kohrman, A., & Munro, C. (1982). Patient characteristics that elicit negative responses from family physicians. *Journal of Family Practice, 14*, 881–882.

Mackway-Jones, K., & Walker, M. (1999). *Pocket guide to teaching for medical instructors.* London: BMJ Books.

Maslow, A. (1954). *Motivation and personality.* New York: Harper & Row.

McGraw, R., & Verma, S. (2001). The trainee in difficulty. *Canadian Journal of Emergency Medicine, 3*, 205–208.

Postman, N., & Weingartner, C. (1969). *Teaching as a subversive activity.* New York: Penguin Education.

Quirk, M. (1994). *How to learn and teach in medical school.* Springfield, IL: Charles C. Thomas.

Robbins, S., & Stuart-Kotze, R. (1990). *Management, concepts and applications.* Englewood Cliffs, NJ: Prentice Hall.

Shapiro, J., Prislin, M., Larsen, K., & Lenahan, P. (1987). Working with the resident in difficulty. *Family Medicine, 19,* 369–375.

Tiberius, R. (1995). *Small group teaching: A trouble-shooting guide.* Toronto: OISE Press/Ontario Institute for Studies in Education.

Evaluation

As the months passed, the medical staff at the Clinics of Main Street were becoming more comfortable with the strategies for teaching their trainees on a day-to-day basis. Dr. Smith had followed the process by periodically asking each of them about their progress.

Several of his colleagues mentioned that they could benefit from having a system to summarize for the trainees all the information that they were gathering on their performance daily. The teachers had amassed considerable data but had no method for gathering all these facts together and reviewing them for the trainees. The staff also wanted to pool the information gathered by several different teachers into one comprehensive report.

Dr. Smith also wanted the trainees to tell him how they thought the doctors were performing as teachers and how the clinic's staff were performing overall as members of a teaching center. Although he had obtained informal comments from the trainees as they finished their rotation, he wanted a detailed, anonymous system that would be more revealing and helpful.

Dr. Smith invited an expert on evaluation from the university's faculty of education to their next evening meeting to show them how an evaluation system could work in their office. Here is what they covered.

WHAT IS EVALUATION?

Evaluation is the guiding instrument of the learner, teacher, and program director. Just as various dials guide an airplane on its flight path, evaluation instruments inform you if you are on course, if there is need for midcourse correction, or if you have reached your destination (Rossi, 1999; Cunnington, Hanna, Turnbull, Kaigas, & Norman, 1997). The destination is predetermined when both you and the trainee establish learning objectives at the outset (Hutchinson, 1999). Evaluation consists of finding out the extent to which each of these objectives has been attained and the quality of teaching techniques and teachers (Snell et al., 2000).

Evaluation for Learners

1. *What to evaluate?* Determine the following before undertaking your trainee's formal evaluation.
    a. Begin with the objectives of the course or rotation as set by the medical school or hospital program. It is important for both the student and the program to know whether the learner has achieved the knowledge, attitudes, and skills expected during the time allotted in your office.
    b. Determine the learner's personal objectives as outlined in any learning plan that you establish with him at the outset (Harborow, 2000).
    c. Evaluate the learner's overall performance for that level of training. Ensure that these objectives have primacy over any particular interest of your own (Bedinghaus & Bragg, 1998).
2. *Who is being evaluated?* Be clear about what level of training the trainees have reached so that you will have appropriate expectations for knowledge and skills. If possible, obtain from the hospital or medical school a summary of the trainees' background and performance to date. It is also useful to ask them at their first session about their academic background. Obtaining information on trainees who have had academic or behavioral difficulties makes it possible to set up special learning objectives (Corley, 1983).
3. *What is the gold standard?* Evaluation works best for both learner and teacher when a gold standard or optimal performance criteria for the various knowledge and skill levels have been established. Ask if the hospital, medical school, and certifying body have them (Liebrandt, Kukora, & Dent, 2001). If not, develop some for your office, and use these as the basis for the trainee's evaluation.

Example: The following are optimal performance criteria for charting (Borgiel et al., 1989):

    a. Chart is legible
    b. Problem-oriented format used

     c.   Patient profile completed on all charts

     d.   Key findings of history and physical included, both positive and negative

     e.   Working diagnosis indicated clearly

     f.   Management plan and follow-up of patient indicated

4.   *When to evaluate?*

     a.   At the beginning of the rotation—Review the course objectives with the trainee and set up a personal learning plan. Outline the evaluation system used at your office and incorporate additional items as necessary from the learning plan. Give the trainee a copy of the evaluation form you use. Distribute any lists of performance criteria you have developed.

     b.   In the middle—Halfway through the rotation or course, complete an interim evaluation with the trainee and modify the learning plan based on identified weaknesses. Known as formative evaluation, this is designed to let the trainee know how far she has progressed in achieving her objectives. The strategies described in chapter 4, such as direct observation and criterion chart review, are other examples of providing specific evaluation to learners during the course of their time with you. They enable learning activities to be modified based on identified strengths and weaknesses to date (Ende, Pomerantz, & Erickson, 1995; Tessmer, 1993).

         It is difficult to provide this formative evaluation because other priorities seem to take precedence in a busy practice. Set an objective for yourself to complete a clinical encounter evaluation form and review it with your trainee once a week. The information is based on your review of a single patient seen by your trainee, selected at random. The regular task of completing the form acts as a stimulus for formative evaluation. Figure 6.1 shows a sample clinical encounter evaluation form.

     c.   At the end—Before the rotation ends, complete the final evaluation. Known as summative evaluation, this informs the trainee whether she has achieved her personal objectives as well as those of the medical school for that course. It should identify areas of knowledge and skills that need to be improved and that could be included in the trainee's next set of learning objectives (Mackway-Jones & Walker, 1999).

         Always meet with the learner in person. Do not leave the evaluation in her mailbox without providing an opportunity for discussion of the details.

Clinics of Main Street
Sample Clinical Encounter Evaluation Form

Name _____ **Date** _____

Scale   4-excellent   3- good   2- fair   1-poor   N/A-not applicable

Item	Score	Comments
• History		
• Physical		
• Investigation		
• Treatment		
• Patient education		
• Prevention		
• Organization		
• Presentation		
• Documentation		

Comments on strengths and weaknesses

_____

_____

_____

_____

_____

Supervisor's signature _____

Student's signature _____

FIGURE 6.1   Sample Clinical Encounter Evaluation Form.

5. *How to evaluate?* The following are ways to evaluate trainees:
    a. Gathering of information—At your regular staff meetings, set aside
        some time for evaluation of the trainees working in the office.
        Have the objectives for each trainee's rotation available as well as
        each learning plan. Ask each staff member who has worked with
        the trainee for individual details. Usually one staff member has
        overall responsibility for the trainees. Have this person take notes
        of the comments and transfer them to the evaluation sheet (Beach,
        McCormick, & Levine, 1991).
    b. Promotion of self-evaluation—Once trainees have left formal train-
        ing programs and entered practice, they must assess their own
        strengths and weaknesses to guide their continuing education.
        You can enhance this skill by asking the trainees to complete the
        evaluation form for themselves before attending the session when
        you review the staff comments with them. By looking at themselves
        and comparing their evaluation to what others think, they will
        get some insight into the accuracy of their self-image (Hodges,
        Regeher, & Martin, 2001; Ward, Gruppen, & Regeher, 2002).
    c. Sample form—When completing the form, remember the guide-
        lines for providing information to learners on their performance
        (chapter 2). These principles are as applicable to formal evaluation
        as to the one-on-one situation. Ensure that you conclude the evalu-
        ation with some general recommendations to guide the student's
        future learning (Corley, 1983).

Figure 6.2 shows a sample student evaluation form.

EVALUATION FOR TEACHERS

It is important to review and improve your teaching skills periodically.
The most helpful source of information on your present skills are comments
from trainees working in your office (Skeff, 1988; Stritter, Baker, & McGahie, 1983). You can gather informal impressions of your teaching skills
from the trainees by asking them to comment about their learning experiences. Some trainees have the confidence to give you direct comments on
your role in their learning. For most trainees, it is a difficult task, because
they fear being disliked afterward and also fear a negative influence on
their final evaluation. A less confrontational approach is to have trainees
complete an anonymous teacher evaluation form, preferably after their
evaluation is completed (Skett, Campbell, & Stratos, 1984).

CLINICS OF MAIN STREET

SAMPLE STUDENT EVALUATION FORM

NAME _____ DATE _____

Scale 5 - excellent 4 - good 3 - fair 2 - poor 1 - failure

Item	Score	Comments
• Information gathering (history, physical exam, investigation)		
• Manual skills (diagnostic tests, minor surgery, office procedures)		
• Knowledge (identify problems, fund of knowledge, clinical acumen)		
• Problem solving (identify issues, generate hypotheses)		
• Decision making ability (decisions regarding investigation and treatment)		
• Critical thinking (assess evidence skillfully)		
• Attitude to patients (see patient as whole person and consider social and psychological dimensions)		
• Professional responsibility (integrity, reliability, initiative, dependability)		
• Work in groups (relationships with medical staff, office staff, consultants, peers)		
• Self directed learning ability (ability to recognize weaknesses, set learning strategies and achieve objectives)		
• Overall assessment (clinical competence as physician)		

SUMMARY

Strengths	Weaknesses

General Comments _____
_____
_____
_____

Supervisor's signature _____ Student's signature _____

FIGURE 6.2 Sample Student Evaluation Form.

Development of Teacher Evaluation Form

The typical teacher evaluation form lists several characteristics of teaching, usually in the positive mode, and asks for the students' rating and any comments on these points. The attributes evaluated should bear some relationship to the theory you use to guide your daily instruction. Use a faculty meeting to gather a list of criteria that all would consider important for evaluation. This way, everyone knows what is being evaluated by the trainees. When choosing the characteristics, remember that the goal of the form is to help you all set a plan for improving your teaching skills by identifying any remediable weaknesses (Irby, Ramsey, & Gillmore, 1991).

Based on the theory in chapters 1 and 2, a selection from the following list of teaching characteristics could be used.

Individual Qualities

- Enthusiasm
- Approachability
- Confidence
- Empathy, warmth, and affability
- Organization
- Interest in student as a person
- Openness to student comments

Teaching Skills

- Adapts to student's needs and level
- Uses a variety of teaching skills and questioning
- Challenges learner beyond existing level
- Encourages student responsibility in learning
- Promotes learner self-confidence
- Encourages self-evaluation
- Provides learner-based information that is specific and clear
- Stimulates learner to be active and to ask questions
- Assists learner to formulate learning objectives

Learning Environment

- Is a satisfactory role model
- Provides ample opportunity to apply new knowledge and skills

- Establishes comfortable learning setting: space, chairs, light, time
- Establishes a collegial relationship with trainees
- Uses learner knowledge as valid basis for learning
- Sets mutually determined goals of learning as well as strategies to reach goals
- Sets case mix and teaching that are consistent with objectives of program and student's personal learning plan
- Is readily available for advice
- Uses other learners as sources of information (Kernan & O'Connor, 1997)

Figure 6.3 shows a sample teacher evaluation form.

What to Do with the Information: The following indicate applications of this information:

- Each teacher should review the forms after they have been completed by the trainees.
- The teacher can look for ways of learning new teaching skills based on the information or discuss the forms with the clinic director or program director at the associated hospital or medical school (Brinko, 1993).
- As a group, the staff could use the information to plan a teaching skills session at a faculty meeting.

EVALUATION FOR THE TEACHING CENTER

Finally, you want to know what your trainees think of your office as a teaching center.

Figure 6.4 shows a sample teacher center evaluation form.

What to Do with This Information: The clinic director should review each form and see if there are any significant trends that require further investigation. A summary of the comments (both positive and negative) as well as any potentially valuable suggestions should be presented at a staff meeting. Methods of improving on weak areas can be formally discussed at an evening faculty session.

PITFALLS IN EVALUATION

From our experience, the following are the most common hazards in evaluation:

CLINICS OF MAIN STREET

SAMPLE TEACHER EVALUATION FORM

TEACHER'S NAME _____ DATE _____

Scoring	Agree 5	4	3	2	Disagree 1
INDIVIDUAL QUALITIES					
• enthusiastic					
• approachable					
• confident					
• sympathetic/warm					
• well organized					
• interested in learner as person					
TEACHING SKILLS					
• adaptable					
• uses a variety of teaching skills					
• tells the answers directly					
• shares learning responsibility					
• promotes self-confidence					
• coaches self assessment					
• provides examples to support comments					
• stimulates learner beyond current level					
• attuned to individual learning plan					
• uses questions to help you find answer					
LEARNING ENVIRONMENT					
• excellent role model					
• provides chance to apply new skills					
• sets comfortable space					
• collegial interaction					
• available					

COMMENTS _____
_____
_____
_____
_____

FIGURE 6.3 Sample Teacher Evaluation Form.

CLINICS OF MAIN STREET

SAMPLE TEACHING CENTER EVALUATION FORM

We would appreciate your comments on the learning experience during your time with us. Please complete this form by marking the scale next to each sentence and write in any specific comments below.

Scoring	Agree 5	4	3	2	Disagree 1
■ This experience was appropriate to the curriculum goals of my hospital or medical school					
■ I had the opportunity to establish and apply my own personal learning goals as well					
■ The balance between service and learning was appropriate.					
■ There was a broad spectrum of clincal problems and patients					
■ There was sufficient formal and informal teaching					
■ There was regular comment on my clinical performance					
■ The working facilities provided to me were adequate					
■ I had considerable responsibility for my patient's care.					
■ Overall, I enjoyed this learning experience.					

Indicate the frequency of use of the following:

	never	sometime	often	daily
case discussion				
chart review				
direct observation				
video replay				
tutorials on topics				

Features I would continue or expand _____

_____

_____

Features I would change and how _____

_____

FIGURE 6.4   Sample Teaching Center Evaluation Form.

1. *Failure to evaluate:* Students finish their rotation in your office and leave without receiving any formal evaluation. According to learning theory, students really want to know how they are progressing, always wonder how the teachers rate their performance, and want that information as soon as possible (Krause, 2000).

2. *Halo effect:* The teacher rates everyone at a certain level, usually "good." Alternatively, the teacher scores all categories on a given learner's evaluation form with the same mark (e.g., a student who is particularly good at one task gets all the other items rated highly because of the spillover effect; a student who is particularly unreliable may get all categories rated poorly even though her performance may be quite adequate for some specific items) (Cockayne & Samuelson, 1978). Few trainees perform exceptionally well or badly in every area. They all have different strengths and weaknesses. The teacher must assess each category in and of itself.

3. *Teacher biases:* The teacher who is biased against trainees for whatever reason may allow these prejudices to interfere with an objective assessment.

4. *Reliance on terminal evaluations:* Evaluation should be seen as an ongoing process requiring interaction with trainees at various intervals during the time at your office. One evaluation at the end is helpful, but several evaluations along the way, with suggestions for change, are much more helpful.

5. *Failure to fail:* Teachers are reluctant to identify trainees with considerable difficulty. They try to "pass" students without informing them of their serious misgivings or conveying the information to the medical school or hospital education office.

REFERENCES

Beach, P., McCormick, D., & Levine, H. (1991). Implementation of a mentor system to enhance student education and evaluation in the ambulatory setting. *Teaching and Learning in Medicine, 3,* 151–155.

Bedinghaus, J., & Bragg, D. (1998). Use of behavioural descriptors for performance evaluation in first and second year clinical experience. *Academic Medicine, 73,* 580–582.

Borgiel, A., Williams, I., Bass, M., Evenson, M., Lamont, C., MacDonald, P., McCoy, M., & Spasoff, R. (1989). Quality of care in family practice: Does residency training make a difference? *Canadian Medical Association Journal, 140,* 1035–1043.

Brinko, K. (1993). The practice of giving feedback to improve teaching. What is effective? *Journal of Higher Education, 64,* 574–593.

Cockayne, T., & Samuelson, C. (1978). Halo effect and medical student evaluation of instruction. *Journal of Medical Education, 53*, 364.

Corley, J. (1983). *Evaluating residency training* (2nd ed.). Lexington, MA: Collamore Press.

Cunnington, J., Hanna, E., Turnbull, J., Kaigas, T., & Norman, G. (1997). Defensible assessment of the competency of the practicing physician. *Academic Medicine, 72,* 9–12.

Ende, J., Pomerantz, A., & Erickson, F. (1995). Preceptors' strategies for correcting residents in an ambulatory care medicine setting. *Academic Medicine, 70,* 224–229.

Harborow, P. (2000). Personal learning plan and mentoring. *Education for General Practice, 11,* s512–514.

Hodges, B., Regeher, G., & Martin, D. (2001). Difficulties in recognizing one's own incompetence: Novice physicians who are unskilled and unaware of it. *Academic Medicine, 76,* s87–89.

Hutchinson, L. (1999). Evaluating and researching the effectiveness of educational interventions. *British Medical Journal, 318,* 1267–1269.

Irby, D. (1983). Evaluating instruction in medical education. *Journal of Medical Education, 58,* 844–849.

Irby, D., Ramsey, P., & Gillmore, G. (1991). Characteristics of effective clinical teachers of ambulatory care medicine. *Academic Medicine, 66,* 54–55.

Kernan, W., & O'Connor, P. (1997). Site accommodations and preceptor behaviours valued by 3rd year students in ambulatory internal medicine clerkships. *Teaching and Learning in Medicine, 9,* 96–102.

Krause, K. (2000). Formative feedback. In P. Paulman, J. Susman, & C. Abboud (Eds.), *Precepting medical students in the office.* Baltimore: Johns Hopkins University Press.

Liebrandt, T., Kukora, J., & Dent, T. (2001). Integrating educational objectives and the evaluation process in a general surgery residency program. *Academic Medicine, 76,* 748–752.

Mackway-Jones, K., & Walker, M. (1999). *Pocket guide to teaching for medical instructors.* London: BMJ Books.

Rossi, P. (1999). *Evaluation: A systematic approach.* Thousand Oaks, CA: Sage Publishing.

Skeff, K. (1988). Enhancing teaching effectiveness and vitality in the ambulatory setting. *Journal of General Internal Medicine, 3,* S526–533.

Skeff, H., Campbell, M., & Stratos, G. (1984). Evaluation of attending physicians: Three perspectives. *Proceedings of the 23rd Annual Conference on Research in Medical Education, 23,* 277–281.

Snell, L., Tallett, S., Haist, S., Hays, R., Norcini, J., Prince, K., Rothman, A., & Rowe, R. (2000). A review of the evaluation of clinical teaching: New perspectives and challenges. *Medical Education, 34,* 862–870.

Stritter, F., Baker, R., & McGahie, W. (1983). Congruence between residents' and clinical instructors' perception of teaching in outpatient care center. *Medical Education, 17,* 385–389.

Tessmer, M. (1993). *Planning and conducting formative evaluations.* London: Kogan Page.

Ward, M., Gruppen, L., & Regeher, G. (2002). Measuring self-assessment. *Advances in Health Sciences Education, 7,* 63–80.

Index